YOGA
IN THE WORKPLACE

Shameem Akthar is a certified yogacharya trained with the Sivananda Yoga Vedanta Center, Kerala. A columnist with several prestigious publications like *Mid-day*, *India Abroad*, Rediff.com, *Savvy* and *Life Positive*, she teaches and holds workshops related to yoga in Mumbai where she lives with her husband Saisuresh Sivaswamy and daughter Jahnavi Sheriff.

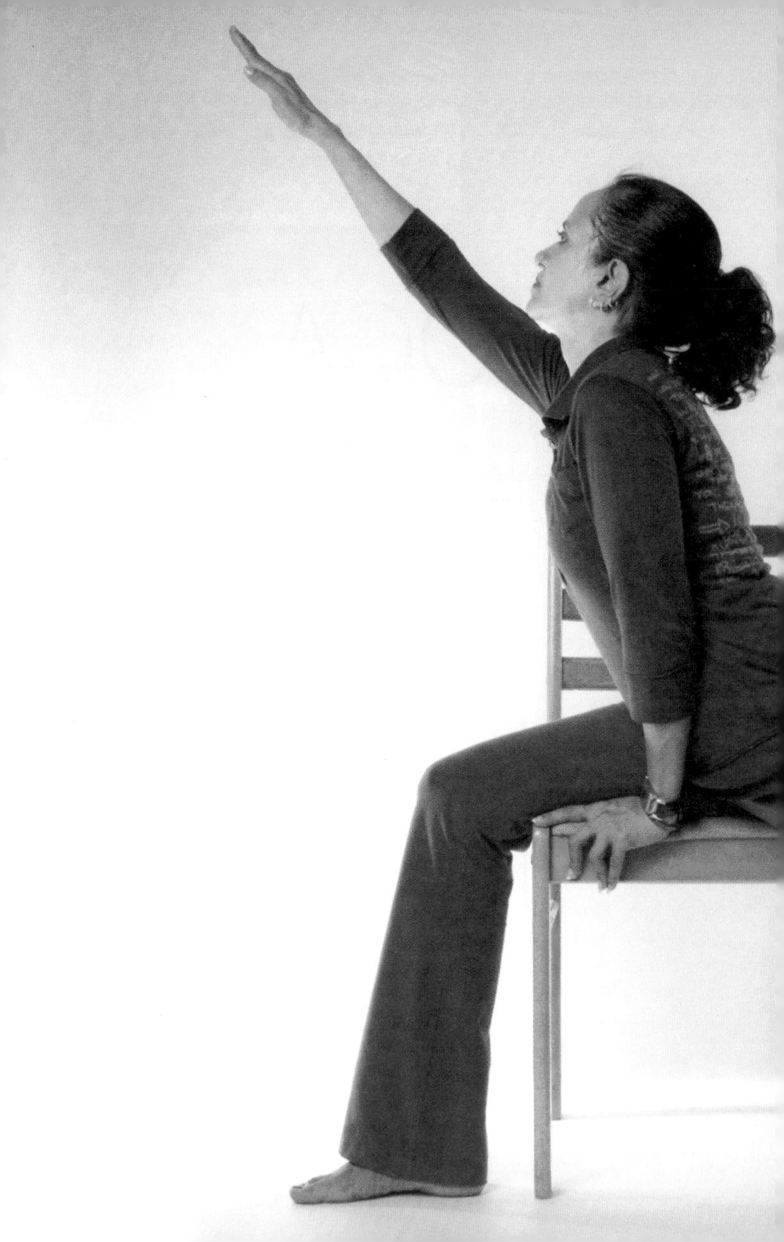

Shameem Akthar

YOGA

IN THE WORKPLACE

westland ltd
Venkat Towers, 165, P. H. Road, Maduravoyal, Chennai 600 095
No.38/10 (New No.5), Raghava Nagar,
New Timber Yard Layout, Bangalore 560 026
Survey No. A - 9, II Floor, Moula Ali Industrial Area,
Moula Ali, Hyderabad 500 040
23/181, Anand Nagar, Nehru Road, Santacruz East, Mumbai 400 055
47, Brij Mohan Road, Daryaganj, New Delhi 110 002

First published by westland ltd 2010

10 9 8 7 6 5 4 3 2 1

ISBN: 978-93-80032-82-5

Consult your doctor before beginning any new exercise programme. The author and publishers assume no responsibility for injuries suffered while practicing these techniques. If you are elderly or have any chronic or recurring conditions such as high blood pressure, neck or back pain, arthritis, heart disease, seek your doctor's advice before practicing.

Design: design-on-u

Printed at Manipal Press Ltd., Manipal

Model credits : The author Shameem Akthar was assisted by her daughter Jahnavi Sheriff.

CONTENTS

At a loose end after my first book, I wrote to Tariq Ansari, the dynamic publisher of Mid-Day Publications, asking if I could expand on my weekly capsules on office yoga for his newspaper, into a book for them. He reluctantly responded that a book was not on his agenda just then. The same week Subashree Krishnaswamy called on behalf of Westland Ltd, asking me for a list of book ideas, and office yoga was one among several I sent. She, as well as the publishers, liked this idea the best. This is, therefore, a book that was meant to be.

If you are reading this book, then you are part of that energy loop of some things that are meant to be. A loop which reaches right back to my Sadguru Swami Sivananda, since for me, everything I do is a gift from my Sadguru—whether it be my own personal practice, asana jaya or victory over a yoga pose, or my own yoga writings. If a gift can also be an offering, then this book is both.

ACKNOWLEDGEMENTS

I thank my asana guru Prahlada for infecting me with his superlative energy and amazing grace as a teacher. This book is an attempt at imitation: trying to copy his stupendous energy and givingness as a teacher. His ability to multi-task, yet retain a cheerful buoyancy of spirit is what I wish to copy and had tried to, while compiling this book.

Though some of the practices are existing classical ones, most others had to be rethought and reset in an office atmosphere. Many practices are created or adapted exclusively for this book.

Here, I also wish to thank all those media editors who had the guts to promote yoga writing when it was a far cry from the fad it has become today: this includes Andrea Costabir (*Savvy*), Meenal Baghel (both when she was with *Mid-Day*, and now as editor of *Mumbai Mirror*), Suma Verghese (*Life Positive*), Meeta Bhatti (*Harmony* magazine), Tinaz Nooshian (Life@work section, *Mid-Day*), Archana Pai (*New Woman*), Nikhil Lakshman (Rediff.com and India Abroad), N. Radhakrishnan (*MansWorld*), Yeshwant Vyas (*Aha Zindagi*), Praveen Chopra (former editor of *Life Positive*). Their support has been an invaluable part of who I am as a yoga writer today.

Last but not the least, my husband Saisuresh Siva swamy and daughter Jahnavi Sheriff, who complement my love for yoga by participating in its magic too.

FOREWORD

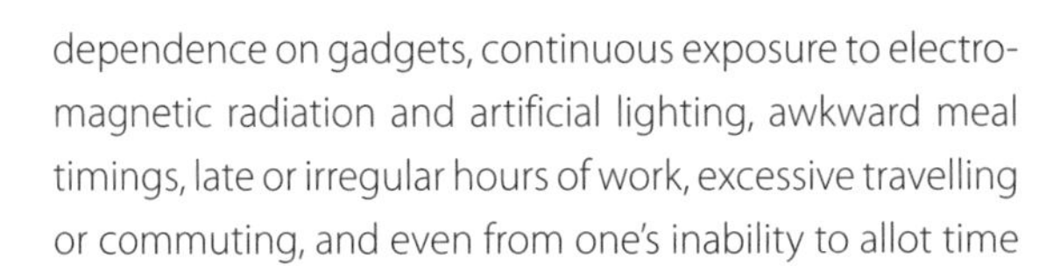

Ancient texts describe yoga as a union between the divine soul and the ordinary self. Today we know it simply as the coordination between our body and our mind. We no longer need to think of yoga as something done exclusively by those who reside in the caves of the Himalayas. Our ancient yogis had created such a powerful tool that it could be, and is still being used effectively to deal with modern-day stress and strain, emanating from demanding jobs and hectic lifestyles.

Yoga teaches us the ability to delve deeper into our minds to examine our reactions to life's challenges. This clarity helps us take on the pounding of daily life, so that we are able to remain positive and optimistic, come what may.

Stress is not just a creation of the mind. Often, it is created by lifestyle changes: a sedentary job, excessive dependence on gadgets, continuous exposure to electro-magnetic radiation and artificial lighting, awkward meal timings, late or irregular hours of work, excessive travelling or commuting, and even from one's inability to allot time for exercise. All or any of these factors can wreak havoc on our health.

Taking all the above factors into consideration, my student Shameem Akthar has come up with a simple and efficient way of using yogic practices wherever you are — at the work station or in your kitchen. These adapted yogic practices can be neatly integrated into your work and family environment. They demand very little in terms of time, yet promise to infuse you with health, both mentally and physically.

I consider this book an effective companion for both the officer-goer and the homemaker. It comes in handy for all those who have to juggle both these roles seamlessly in today's times.

Prahlada

Prahlada is a senior and direct disciple of Swami Vishnu-Devananda. He trained under Swamiji from a very young age and is currently director of the Sivananda Yoga Vedanta Center in Toronto as well as a Hatha yoga teacher in the teachers' and advanced teachers' training courses conducted worldwide at Sivananda ashrams.

WHY YOGA AT WORK?

'If you don't make time for a little pain now, be prepared for greater pain later on', — a wise saying that makes huge sense in this age of gadget-induced, desk-bound lifestyles.

Our aim is to shake you out of your stupor and make you realise that a lifestyle married to the desk is, in the long-run, more devastating and dangerous than swimming in the proverbial shark-infested waters. We want to prod you out of it gently, along the way showing you some classic yogic poses that have been adapted to a desk-bound lifestyle.

This book has been developed keeping in mind all our workaholic friends who are committed to their work-stations round the clock. However, it works just as well for couch potatoes who never venture out of their drawing rooms and are forever glued to their TV sets. If a sedentary life is your chosen way, we tell you how to create the best workout within that lifestyle.

This, however, doesn't imply that our regular gym-goers have nothing to gain from this book. Research proves that exercise relegated entirely to one part of

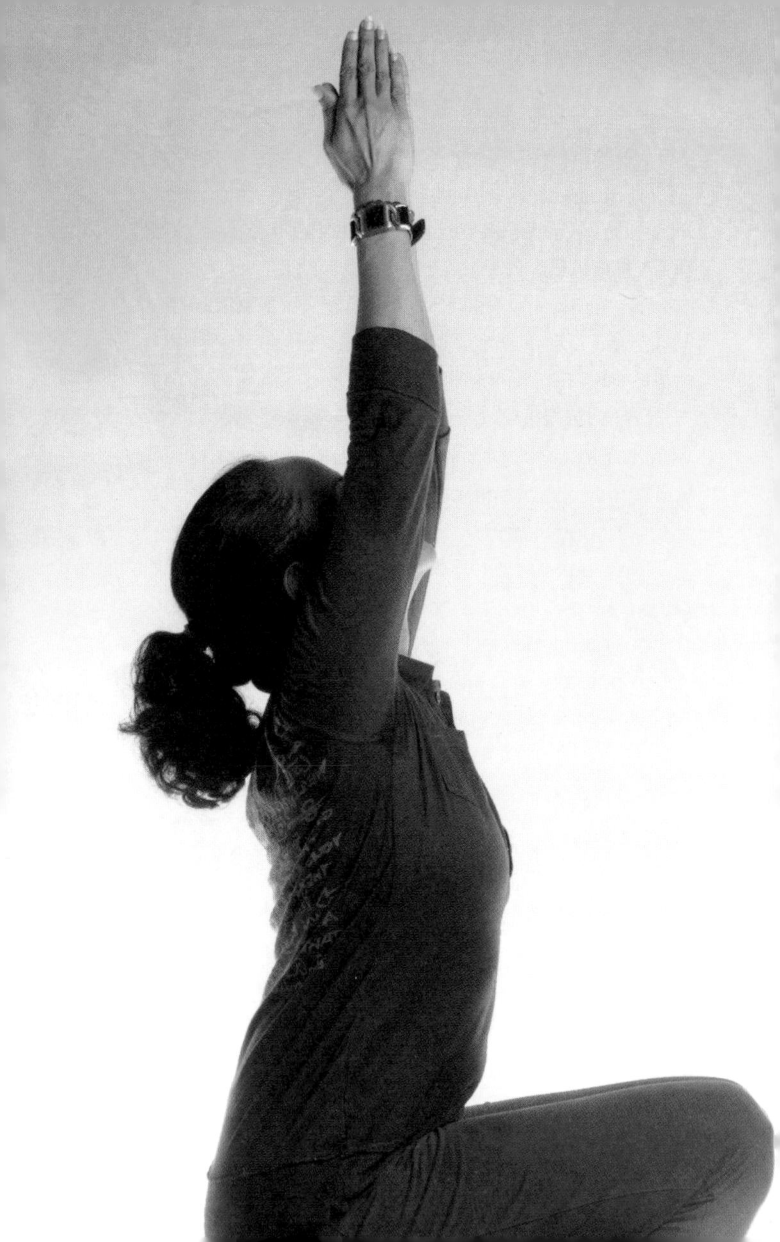

the day is not very effective if the rest of the day is spent largely in a passive manner. This book rectifies that lacuna.

Those who are on their feet for hours at work need to exercise other parts of their bodies throughout the day for long-term health, healing and happiness. Research has established that repetitive activity of a particular body part can cause stress, while disuse of other parts affects the overall health drastically. This is why yoga works the best.

Now, not all offices will encourage their employees to roll out their yoga mats alongside their desks, which is why we show you how to incorporate yoga poses in your daily office routine.

Some of these yogic poses have been around for ages, like the neck circles or agnisara kriya (metabolic fire syndrome); others have been created to accommodate the office environs specifically, without compromising on their effectiveness in the least. It's true that some of these poses can be cumbersome without any proper ground support, like a yoga mat, so you should ideally take a few stretch breaks through the day, and practise those poses that address a specific problem you may have or wish to prevent. For instance, if you are a regular computer user, you need to work on your neck and spine; if you travel regularly, you may wish to focus on the digestive, since eating out regularly has its own hazards that compromise the gut, and ultimately your overall well-being. Keep

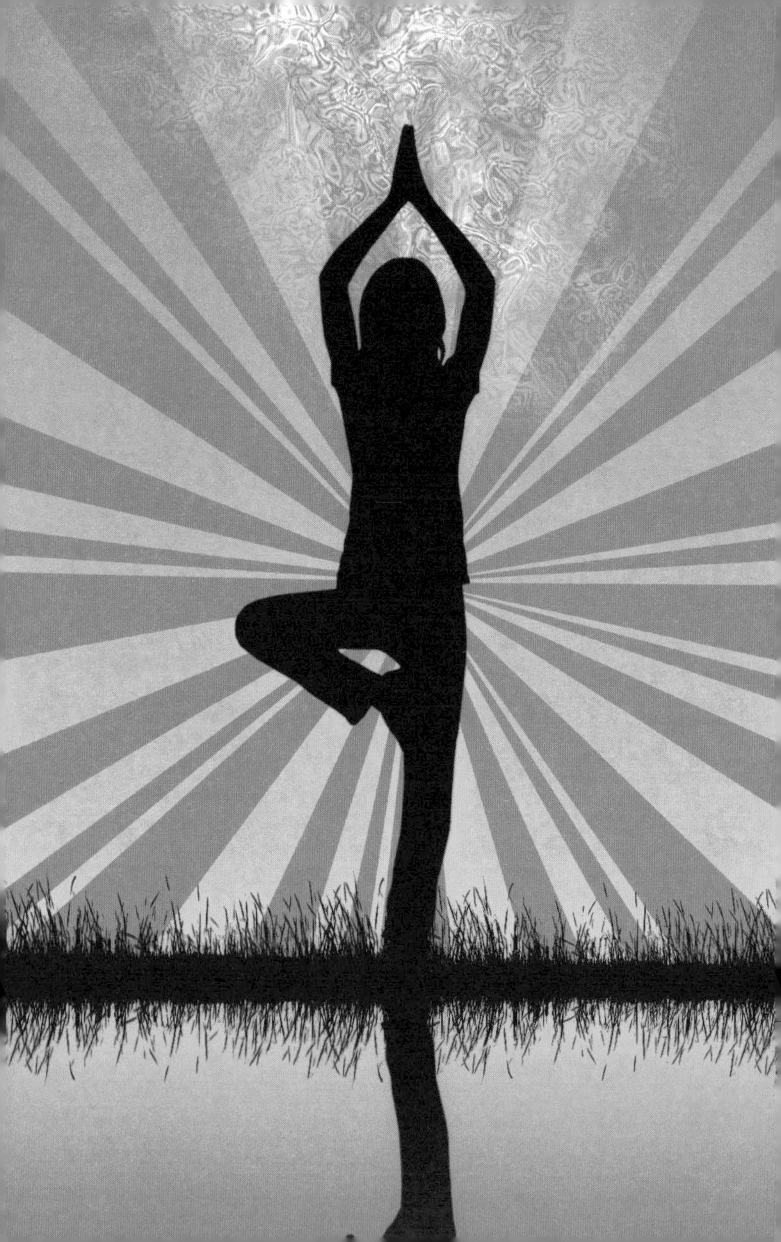

three or four sets of exercises from this book as part of your yoga practice kit. Or, choose one of the charts (at the end of the book) for holistic healing. On days when you feel like skipping office yoga entirely, try and fit in the poses from the short, warm-up yogic stretch chart in your day's schedule.

Allot five minutes of your day to office yoga and see yourself gaining 500 per cent out of it. This is not just another book on yoga — this is about the powerful impact yoga has on your mind and emotional quotient.

So just turn these pages, and allow the book to script a new chapter of your life.

Going ahead with our promise to alarm you, just a bit, about the dangers of a sedentary lifestyle, we bring you this chapter!

The common practice these days, after any chronic ailment or major surgery, is to goad the patient back into some sort of gentle exercise. It has been found that the muscles, bones, and most organs of the body begin to shrivel up after even short-term disuse. In fact, even an exercise freak, after a seven-day gap, will begin to experience a breakdown and loss of all the physical strength he or she has gained. The body constantly renews itself, thus requiring actual motion to ensure transport of repairing agents, nutrients, scarce and rare minerals, blood, oxygen and waste disposal throughout the body. Our body is a living factory. It is unable to work efficiently in a switched-off mode (which is what a sedentary lifestyle is).

SEDENTARY LIFESTYLE =

Below is a list of a few dangers of such a lifestyle:

- Movement is necessary for lymphatic drainage and waste disposal. A quick example would be a clogged drainage system that has not been flushed for a long time.

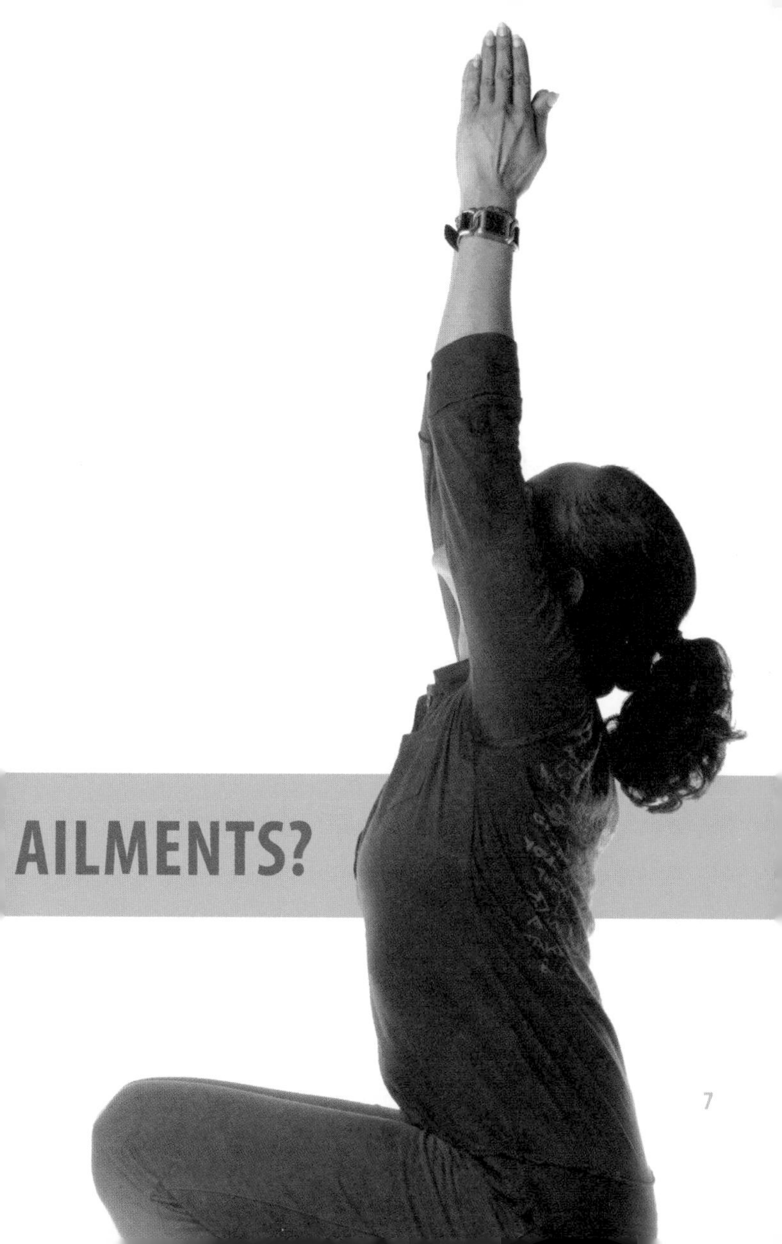

AILMENTS?

- A sedentary lifestyle is almost as bad as smoking, or even worse. If stress is a major trigger in heart problems, a passive way of living is equally to blame in cardiovascular problems, including arteriosclerosis.
- Chronic fatigue syndrome, which accompanies anaemia (iron deficiency), exhaustion, insomnia, lethargy, digestive problems, headaches, non-localised body ache, is caused due to prolonged immobility.
- The new age term 'inactivity stress syndrome' also has similar symptoms.
- Muscle wastes away faster in a passive person. There is a breakdown in muscle protein due to oxidative stress. Which is why a lazy person feels tired after even a simple physical act.
- Bone loss is also faster in a lethargic person. It is an alarming fact that even students, confined to books or passive hobbies, suffer from wrist and hip fractures which used to be common only among the older generation till a few decades ago.
- Bone loss also means the support or foundation under our skin shrinks, causing skin folds and external ageing. A passive person ages faster.
- Internal ageing causes the collapse of all the major systems, including the immune system (which protects against stray and serious infections and

diseases). The immune gland, which actually starts off as the size of an orange when we are infants, begins to shrink alarmingly. But it has been found that an active, focused routine can help regenerate it.

- A sedentary lifestyle might also cause infertility, even as early as in your twenties.
- Remaining inside most of the day, or being exposed to artificial lighting for a long time, can affect sleep patterns. This happens because the pineal gland functions are affected.
- One fallout of this negative impact on the pineal gland, is clinical depression.
- Obesity is another major personal trauma, since fat-to-muscle ratio balloons when you sit around passively. It has been found that excessive fat overturns the body's rhythm, translating into an inbuilt enemy which can manipulate and make important organ systems create toxic and life-threatening conditions. To give you a few examples, it can jeopardise hormonal signals and make excessive fat behave like an independent rogue organ, releasing its own hormones that are on a collision course with the body's natural, health-managing ones.
- Muscle pain, from what is called myofascial pain syndrome, can attack any part of the body. It afflicts mainly those with a sedentary lifestyle.

- A sedentary lifestyle is often accompanied by bad dietary habits (junk food, erratic meals, eating on the run, not chewing food properly to aid digestion, missing meals, eating old/re-heated food, addictions that are regarded as 'harmless' such as excessive intake of coffee, tea or fizzy drinks, etc.), which completely upset the most important flag-bearer of our health — the digestive system. Acidity, reflux, irritable bowel syndrome, constipation, ulcers are just the tip of this disastrous iceberg.
- Chronic insomnia is also common, since movement helps iron out the stress of daily living. And we must not forget that pineal gland connection we spoke of earlier.
- Headaches and migraines are likely to occur due to any of the above given causes.
- Spinal problems, due to the posture a passive lifestyle encourages, are increasingly becoming common even amongst youngsters.
- Oxidative stress is said to be greater amongst passive people. Oxidative stress is also behind that vaguely diagnosed, but alarmingly common, metabolic syndrome, which in turn sets off many chronic ailments. Oxidative stress not only ages us faster, but also hits our health so hard that, not only do we fall ill often, but also recover very slowly.

The list mentioned above is a modest one, so don't be startled just yet. It only gives you a sneak preview into the dangers of a sluggish lifestyle. Awareness of the problem, however, is half the battle won.

To fight the rest of the battle, read on.

Ankle sprains and injuries are extremely common amongst sportsmen. But it isn't their prerogative alone. A person with a sedentary lifestyle is more than likely to fall prey to ankle injury. It is the most common form of injury the world over and, unfortunately, takes the longest time to heal. Even worse, when not properly rehabilitated, it may resurface.

So what are all the possible causes of ankle sprains? Plenty. Squeezing your feet into uncomfortable footwear that does not give stability while walking; lack of exercise; not eating proper meals to support the musculo-skeletal system; and yes, obesity—all these are the culprits. Ankle injuries are not always caused by accidental falls. With sedentary people, the ankle gives way because the muscles supporting the joint have become lazy and flaccid.

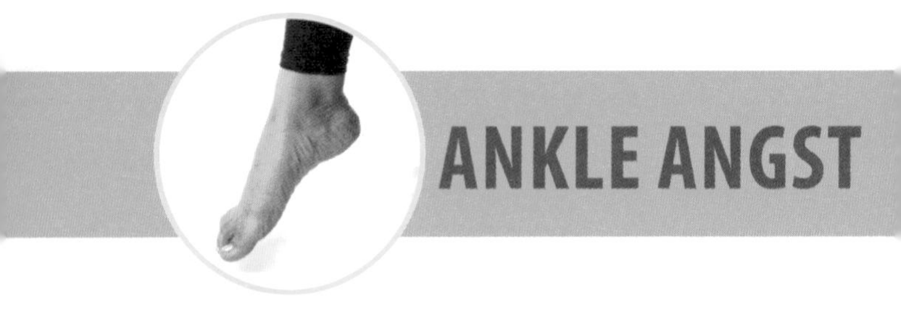

Most people also wrongly assume that walking is a sufficient form of exercise for keeping this overworked and overloaded joint well-lubricated. Of course, walking is better than sitting around. But walking involves only a few sets of muscular challenges. Circles, flexes and extensions are equally necessary to promote the strength of any joint to keep it young. As children we hopped (though, unfortunately, this may not be true of the current generation of kids, which is into passive games and gadgets), skipped and jumped, keeping our ankles strong with these challenges. Apart from maintaining the joints, these games promoted the neuro-muscular co-ordination, thereby creating a healthy link between the brain and the limbs, which facilitated healing.

Here are a few ankle strengthening exercises from yoga, modified so that they can be discreetly done in your office space, or even while travelling.

GOOLF GHOORNAN (ANKLE CRANK)

Method

- Sit on a chair.
- Inhale, point right toe towards the floor (the big toe and the two beside it may touch the floor; the smaller ones will remain off the ground).
- Heel remains raised.
- Adjust right foot so it is straight. Keep it as straight as possible, without straining.
- Continue breathing evenly, holding the pose for a few seconds. This enhances the stretch.
- Release. Rest foot back on the ground. Repeat five to ten times.
- Relax and then repeat for the left foot.

How it works

- The ligaments and tendons that support and work the joint are stretched and strengthened.
- All these exercises challenge the muscles supporting the ankle joint, thus propping it efficiently.

Other benefits

- It works out the entire foot.
- The load-bearing calf muscles are also worked out. They support our posture and weight considerably.

- As observed elsewhere in this book, in reflexology, all our organs have nerve representations in the foot: in effect, these exercises tone our whole body through a shortcut.
- The mind becomes alert, since all feet-leg movements affect the brain through enhanced circulation.

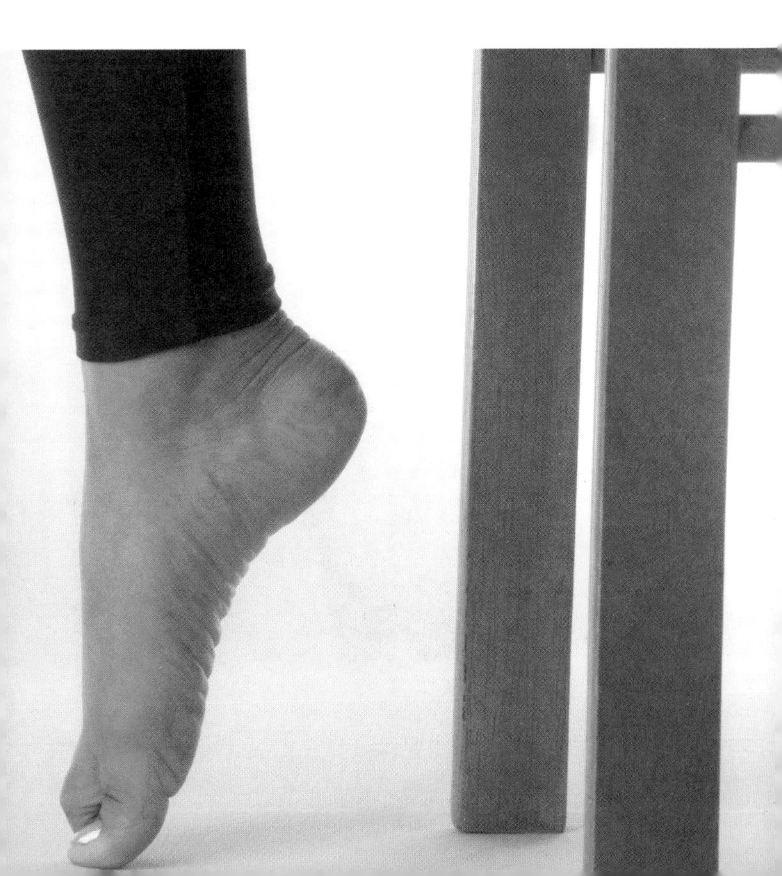

GOOLF GHOORNAN (ANKLE CRANK II)

Method

- Sit on a chair.
- Place right heel on the ground, with an inhalation. Exhale.
- Inhale. Stretch foot at ankle, bending toes backwards, towards yourself.
- Continue breathing evenly. Hold the ankle stretch for a few seconds.
- Release. Rest foot back on the ground. Then repeat five to ten times.
- Relax and then repeat for the left foot.

Benefits

Same as in previous exercise.

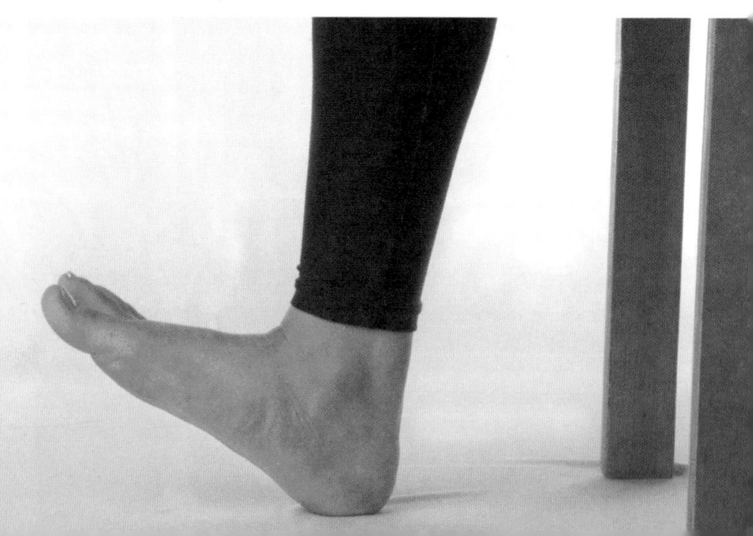

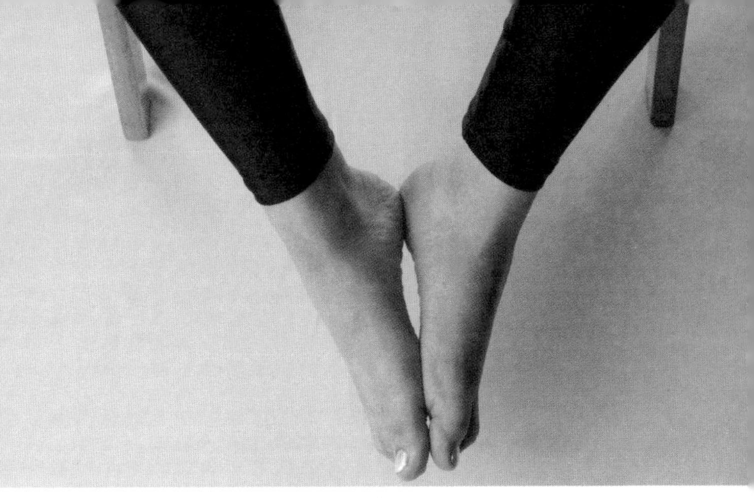

GOOLF NAMAN (ANKLE BEND)

Method

- Sit on a chair.
- Spread knees apart.
- Place soles of both the feet together.
- Adjust, so that all toes are also touching.
- Straighten back. Place palms on either thigh.
- Hold the soles together in this fashion, breathing normally, as long as you can.
- Release, to rest feet back on ground.
- After resting, repeat a few times.

Points to note

- The thighs should be resting on the chair seat. This is important since it may be difficult to hold the feet up otherwise.

- Also, hold only for a few seconds initially. When starting on this exercise, make the first attempt shorter, progressively increasing the duration. Even if doing daily, let the first set be shorter. After the first two times, you may increase the duration.

How it works

- Strengthens the tendons of the ankles, so they can take the pressure of your stride.
- Both legs get a powerful work-out.
- Preventive in any ankle injury.
- Toes are re-trained in the natural art of grip, thus powering your stride and helping to take the load off your ankle.

Other benefits

- Prevents hip injury as well.
- Prevents knee pain.
- Thighs are toned, and become shapely.
- Aids mental focus.
- Feet, which have one of the largest muscle clusters, become elastic and supple.
- Balances both hemispheres of the brain.

GOOLF CHAKRA (ANKLE CIRCLE)

Method

- May be done seated. If done when standing, hold a chair or desk for support. Stand on one leg, for example, on your left leg, bending the right leg at the knee to do this exercise.
- Roll the right ankle in a clockwise direction as if drawing a circle.
- Do this five times.
- Rest foot back on ground.
- Then repeat five rounds in a similar fashion, but drawing a circle with the ankle in an anti-clockwise direction.

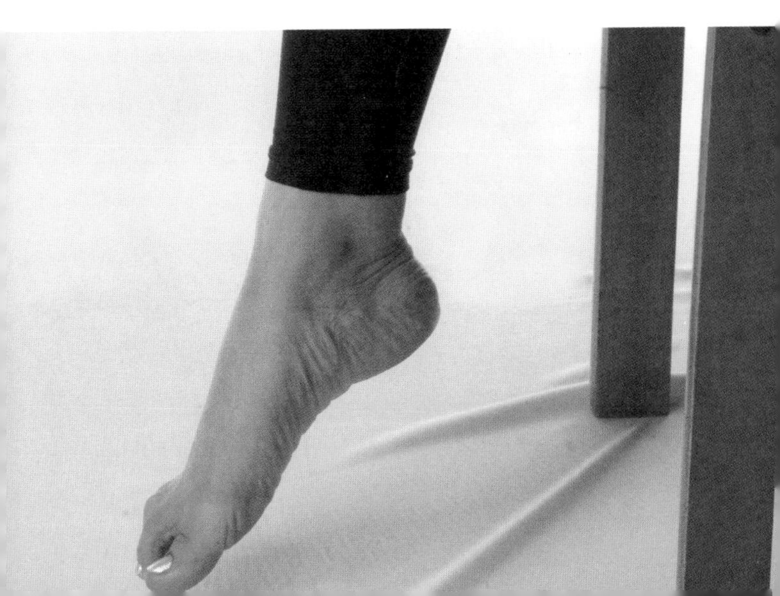

- Rest to repeat the entire sequence for the left leg.
- Breathe normally throughout.

Points to note

- Incorporate breath awareness after a few weeks. Inhale as you begin to draw the circle. Then slowly exhale as you close the circle.
- You may find the left leg is less cooperative. This is because we unconsciously favour the right side in all activity (and vice-versa, for left-handers). So this exercise is a great way to rectify this psycho-physiological make-up.

How it works

- This works the ankle in all directions and is amongst one of the most powerful exercises for ankle health.

Other benefits

- Harmonises both brain hemispheres, creating emotional stability and balance.

TADASANA (PALM TREE POSE)

Method

- To be done standing.
- If your balance is shaky, then stand with your back resting gently against a wall or a strong desk for support. After a few weeks of practice, slowly begin to move away from such props.
- Inhale, raising yourself up on your toes. Remain elevated for five seconds.
- Exhale, lowering the back.
- Inhale, raise yourself now on your heels.
- Hold for five counts. Exhale, to lower the pad of your foot back to the ground.
- This is one round.
- Repeat five to ten rounds.

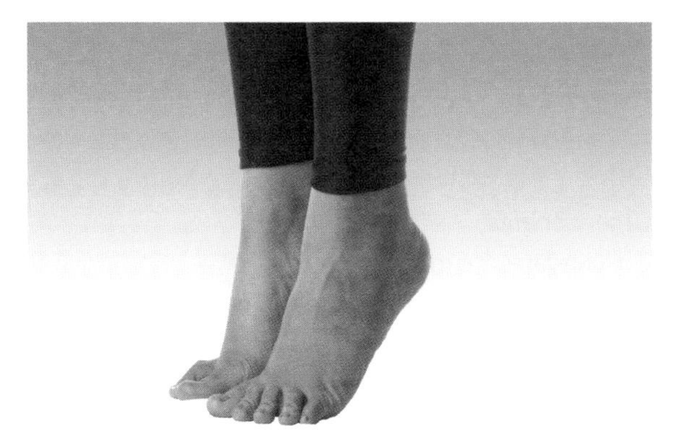

Points to note

You may hold your breath for a few seconds. However, please note that breath retention must be avoided by those suffering from high blood pressure, cardiac ailments or respiratory problems. While holding the breath, lock your stomach muscles when in the final position (on toes or heels). This will help you combine two exercises in one move, plus shape your abdomen, boost metabolism and keep you younger through the stomach lock (uddiyana bandha).

How it works

- Stretches the leg muscles, powering the entire leg, thus propping the ankle well, and taking the body's load off it.
- The joint is also worked well. In fact, a well-worked joint has greater access to nutrients, blood flow, removal of waste and repairing agents.
- This is a powerful resistance trainer that helps the bones in this area become denser and healthier.

Other benefits

- It elevates the mood.
- Increases mental focus by working the leg, which boosts blood flow, including to the heart and brain.
- If you are combining it with the stomach lock, it will increase mental stamina too.

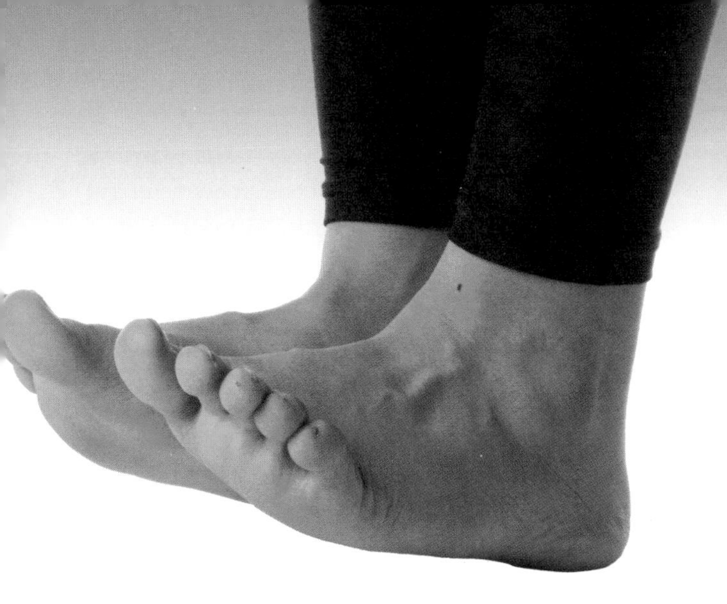

What else?

- An increase in the ability to support body weight also **improves our posture**, since the weight-bearing capacity of the body is fine-tuned.
- All feet-leg workouts impact the brain through improved overall blood circulation. You will begin to enjoy **greater mental clarity**.
- Heart function is also boosted for the above reasons.
- The left-brain hemisphere co-ordination is improved, leading to **mental harmony and equilibrium**.

A bad posture often implies that our feet have lost their natural ability to support our body movements and weight. Usually the reason is bad quality footwear, other than, of course, our passive, chair-bound workstyles. The neglect of one part of the body often shows itself in problems with a different body part. This confounds even medical science. So, neglected feet, bad posture, ill-fitting footwear may, in the long run, be symptomatic of, or cause other problems like back pain, piles and belly fat!

A supple foot has the bounciness to effortlessly carry our weight and the tremendous pressure we exert each time we take a step. The big toe plays a huge role in how we carry ourselves. But all this gets compromised when we don't exercise our feet.

Ever wondered what your air-conditioned surroundings do to your feet? Sitting for a long time in

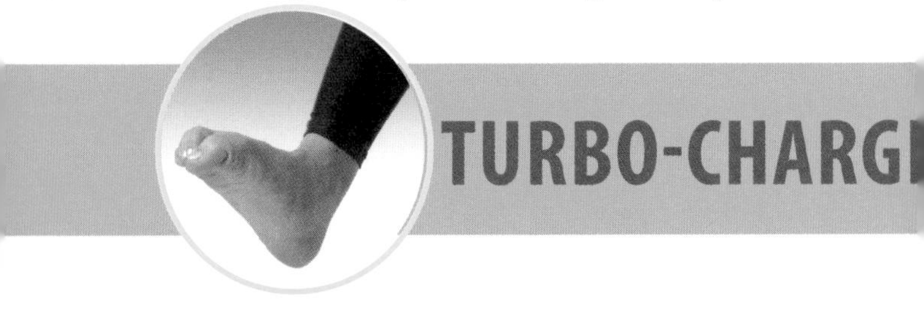

an air-conditioned office causes dehydration. The loss of fluids, in turn, causes the feet to swell up, as the fluid balance in the body goes off kilter.

Sadly, though our feet contain over one-fourth of the total number of bones in the entire body, as well as the maximum number of sweat glands and the highest concentration of nerve endings, they suffer the most neglect and abuse. Below are more dangers when you neglect your feet or fail to appreciate its connection to the other parts of the body:

- In long-haul flights, those with cardiovascular problems often suffer or become victims of a heart attack if they sit in one place for too long (due to embolism: when the emboli originates in the leg and moves to the lung or heart, causing a blockage). Thus leg movement is essential to keep the heart free of such attacks.
- Being indoors, confined to artificial lighting for a long time, affects our body's capacity to manufacture Vitamin D, needed for calcium absorption. Due to this,

unabsorbed calcium deposits are known to lodge in the body. Painful heel spurs that cause excruciating pain can be related directly to this.
- Eating packaged food simply means you are overloading the liver, which must work extra hard

to detox the preservatives used in such items. This means more of the harmful hippuric acid. And where does it accumulate? The feet, especially the toes!

- Similarly, excessive meat consumption means more uric acid. And more deposits in the feet.
- Too much caffeine, tea or cocoa? Or any other form of diuretic? Again, oxalic acid released as metabolic waste finds its way to the feet.
- Even safe fluids, like juices, if made from dubious water sources, could contain solvents which cause these painful deposits.
- Excess salt, sodium (from packaged foods, canned stuff) are also culprits.
- Other culprits include laxatives, contraceptive pills or other hormonal supplements. Not to forget that infamous habit of this generation — excessive pill-popping as a quick-fix for all ailments.

When our clean-up organs or glands like the kidney or liver suffer—due to any of the many abuses listed above—our feet indicate the distress of the whole body by swelling up. In eastern therapies, every part of our body contains a hologram of the entire system. So, neglecting the toes or abusing them (with bad footwear or lack of exercise) could seriously compromise our overall health in the long run.

The following adaptations of classic yogic postures focus on more than just your feet.

PADANGULI NAMAN (TOE STRETCH)

Method

- May be done both standing and sitting.
- Extend your right leg out.
- Now press toes down firmly. Relax.
- Curl toes inwards.
- Do this five to ten times.
- Factor in breath awareness, inhaling while curling the toes inwards and exhaling while pressing them down.
- Rest your foot on the ground for a few seconds.
- Then repeat for the other foot.

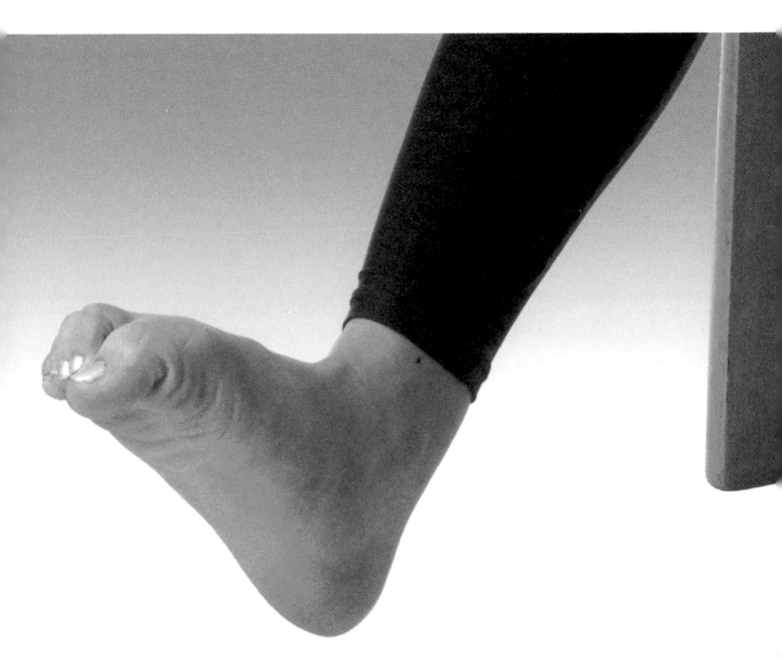

How it works

- This stretches the entire foot, working out tendons, muscles, ligaments.
- Relieves oedema, or swelling of feet, by encouraging blood circulation here.
- Working out the toes gives a better grip to the feet, facilitating movement and perfecting your posture.

Other benefits

- Helps stabilise blood pressure.
- Improves blood flow to the heart by mobilising venous drainage.
- Promotes lymphatic drainage.
- Improves mental alertness when done with breath awareness.

PADANGULI NAMAN (TOE WORKOUT, USING BALL)

Method

- Sit on a chair.
- Place feet slightly apart.
- Place a ball between the feet.
- Try to lift it with both feet.
- Hold it for a few seconds, breathing normally.
- Repeat several times during the day.

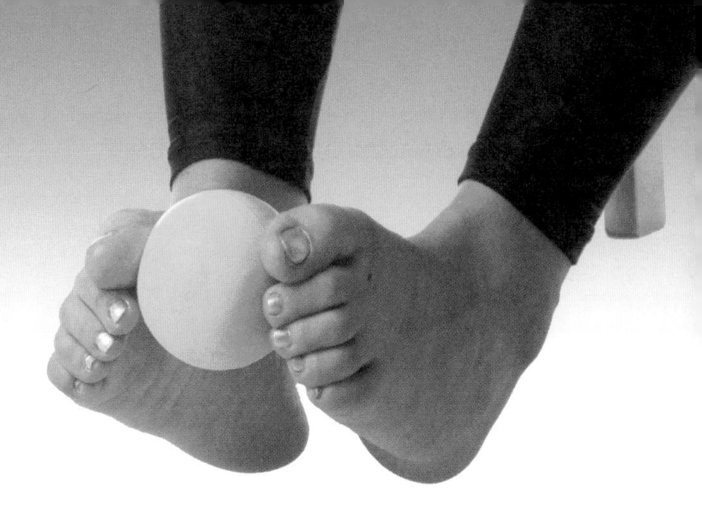

Points to note

You may use any other object other than a ball, but the curves of a ball make the entire task more challenging, thus adding to the workout. This also unleashes a sharper sense of playfulness.

How it works

- It prevents blood pooling at the feet.
- The toes are worked out, making the foot's load-bearing ability more efficient.

Other benefits

- It is a quick emotional pick-me-up.

PADANGULI NAMAN (TOE WORKOUT, USING MARBLE)

Method

- Sit on a chair.
- Place feet slightly apart.
- Place a marble (or something small, like an eraser or even a pen) on the floor.
- Attempt to lift it with your toes.
- Repeat for each foot, for equal workout.

Points to note

This is a little difficult, so the mind is more engaged, giving it a break from the monotony of work. This helps you return to work with more verve.

Benefits

Same as previous exercise.

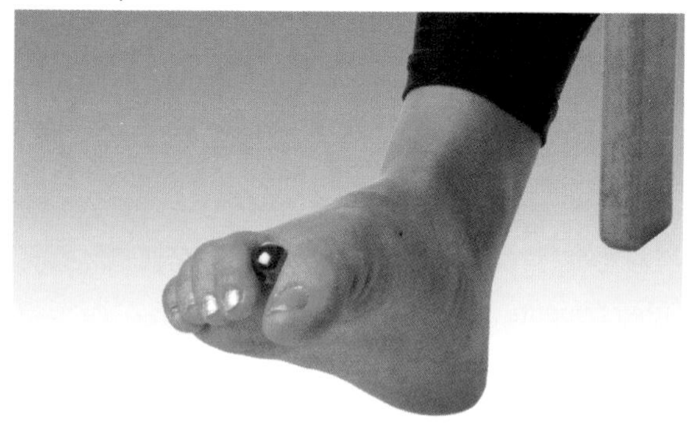

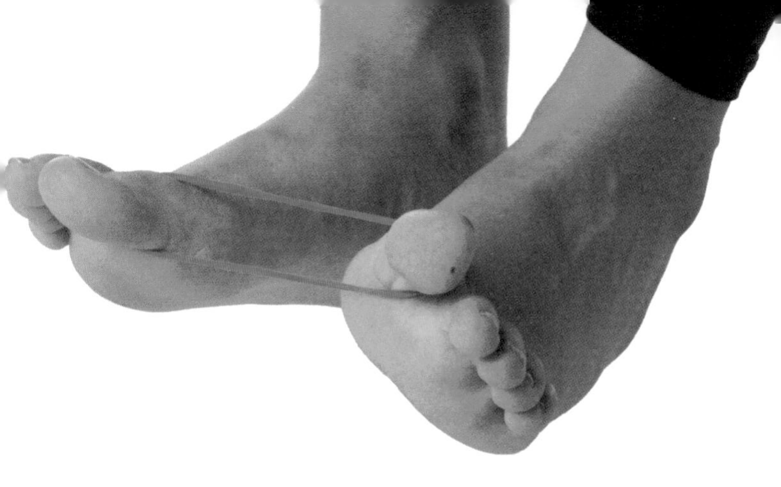

PADANGULI NAMAN (TOE STRETCH, USING A BAND)

Method

- Always done seated.
- Place a strong band (rubber or hair band or even a tie) over the big toes.
- Inhale. Exhaling, stretch the band.
- Hold the stretch to a count of four.
- Release.
- Repeat a few times.

How it works

- Works out the big toe.
- Several important nerve tracts pass through each foot. They are re-trained by this exercise.
- It encourages foot alignment.

Other benefits

Rectifies postural defects.

PADANGULI NAMAN (TOE BENDING, ADVANCED VERSION)

Method

- Sit on a chair.
- Lift your right foot a little off the ground.
- Write a few imaginary alphabets or words in the air with your right foot.
- Do it for a few seconds.
- Repeat for left foot.

Points to note

- Some of you may find that it is difficult to coordinate one foot as well as you do the other. Focus so that you do the weaker foot with greater care and awareness.
- Remember to do an equal number of letters or characters with each foot, so each is equally worked. This also keeps the mind occupied, creating better focus.

How it works

- Works out the entire foot powerfully.
- The grip of the toes, never exercised before, is enhanced.

Other benefits

- This helps align posture by ensuring both feet are bearing your weight equally.
- Encourages playfulness and right brain activation.
- Helps harmonise both brain hemispheres, so our emotional and logical selves are in a state of equilibrium.

What else?

- Working out any part of the lower limb encourages you to think out of the box. It has been found that lower limb movement and **brain cell regeneration** are somehow linked. So work those feet to exercise your grey cells.
- In reflexology, all major systems of our body are related to the foot.

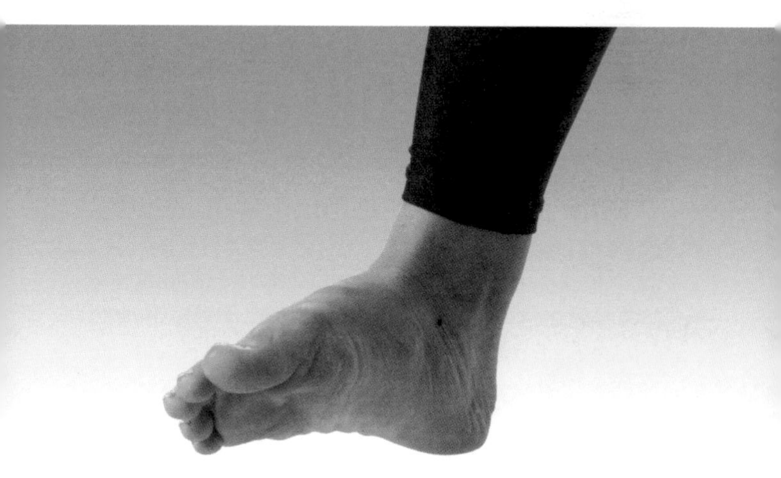

The shoulder is one of the most overworked body parts. Also, the bio-engineering of the shoulder joint demands high maintenance. The main culprit is the shorter muscle-to-bone ratio of this joint. Inactivity or lack of exercise can further shorten the muscle, stiffening the joint. On the other extreme, activities that overextend it, like some sports and hobbies, also ruin it. Keeping it healthy could well mean a difference between immobility and youthful freedom.

Louise L. Hay, motivational healer and seminar leader, says our shoulders represent our ability to withstand the burdens in life. In the opinion of such mind-body therapists, whether we bear our life's burdens with grace or suffering, could decide the difference between pain in the shoulder or a strongly-lubricated joint.

SHOULDERING IT

Intriguingly, shoulder pain could also be symptomatic of an acute cardiac condition. Spine experts also use it to trace neck pain. In certain cases, it could even indicate ailments in the gall bladder or liver. Again, weak shoulders, caused through bad posture, can severely limit our breathing. This means a variety of problems that affect all major systems, including immunity.

But the direct attack on your shoulder joint comes from something over which you definitely have control — your posture.

Sitting hunched up, or slouching in your chair could lead to inflammation of the shoulder muscles or tendons. Even resting your elbows for too long on the arm rests of your chair could cause this pain which is particularly excruciating. What's worse, the pain hits mostly when one is sleeping. This should be of particular concern to those who hold desk-bound jobs.

Since such inactivity means slack muscles, it incapacitates us for simple day-to-day activities like lifting luggage, carrying loads, and indulging in weekend sports, because it increases our chances of suffering a shoulder injury.

Those who love activities like swimming, gardening, ball games or painting are likely to overextend their joint in one particular direction, causing what is called impingement syndrome, a painful inflammation by which the joint expresses an acute distress. Keeping the shoulder joints flexed and working out the supporting muscles with the following yogic postures will ensure that one of the most important parts of our body remains healthy and strong, so we can take on life's challenges with ease.

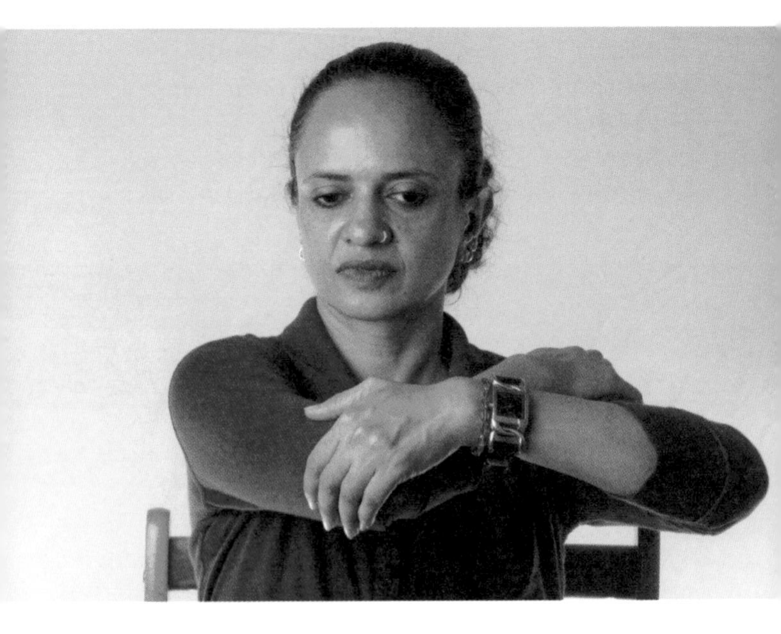

KEHUNI NAMAN (ELBOW BEND)

Method

- May be done seated or standing.
- Place right hand on left shoulder, cupping it.
- Hold right elbow with left hand, cupping it. Inhale.
- Raise both elbows in air, so they are held at chest level.
- Exhale. Using left hand, drag the right elbow across the chest firmly but gently.
- Inhale, releasing the hold.
- Repeat entire sequence five times.
- Repeat the exercise for the opposite side.

How it works

- Provides powerful workout for the entire hand.
- Entire upper body gets a thorough workout.
- Prevents neck pain, stiff shoulder.

Other benefits

- Removes body stiffness and related lethargy.
- Boosts mental alertness.
- Ups respiratory capacity.
- Boosts immunity.

KEHUNI NAMAN (ELBOW BENDING, ADVANCED)

Method

- Repeat the first four steps given in the previous exercise. Inhale.
- Here you must resist the hold of the left hand with your right elbow, exerting opposing pressure from the two hands.
- Hold this for four counts.
- If you do not have cardiac problems or high blood pressure, while holding for four counts, you may also retain your breath.
- Exhale, to release hold.
- Repeat entire sequence five times.
- Release. Relax.
- Repeat for the other side.

Points to note

This can be tough since a greater exertion is called for. Introduce it a few weeks after you start on the first one, especially if you don't exercise regularly. Those used to an active lifestyle may incorporate it earlier.

How it works

Same as previous exercise, though the benefits are more enhanced.

Other benefits

- Breath retention while holding the final pose further expands lung capacity.
- It also impacts the mind, strengthening will-power.

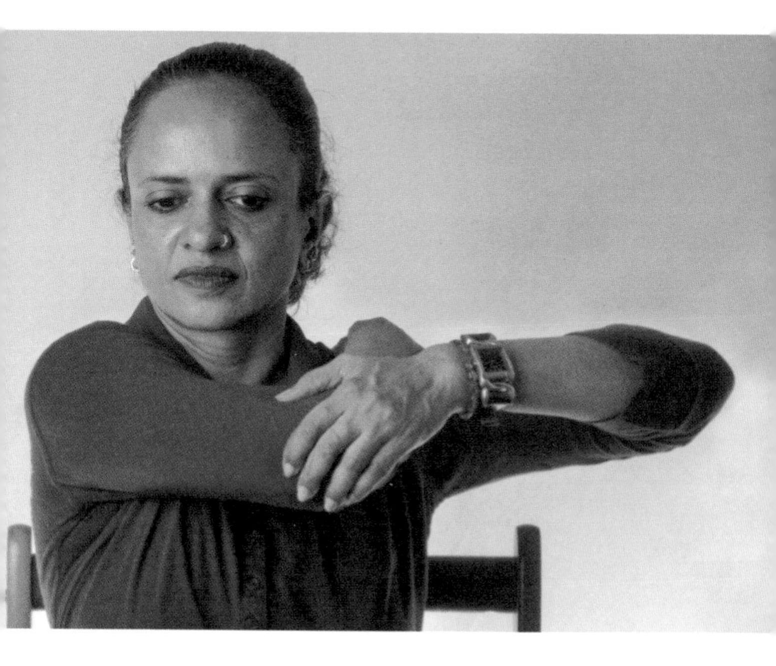

PRANAMASANA (PRAYER POSE)

Method

- May be done seated or standing.
- Inhale, placing palms together in a 'namaste' gesture.
- Exhale, touch the length of the arms together, from fingers to elbow.
- Inhale, raising the hands in this fashion, so the elbows are at face-level.
- Hold the pose, breathing normally.
- Exhale, drop hands down to starting position. Repeat three to five times.

Points to note

If your body is stiff you may not be able to raise your arms too high, so initially raise them only as much as you can.

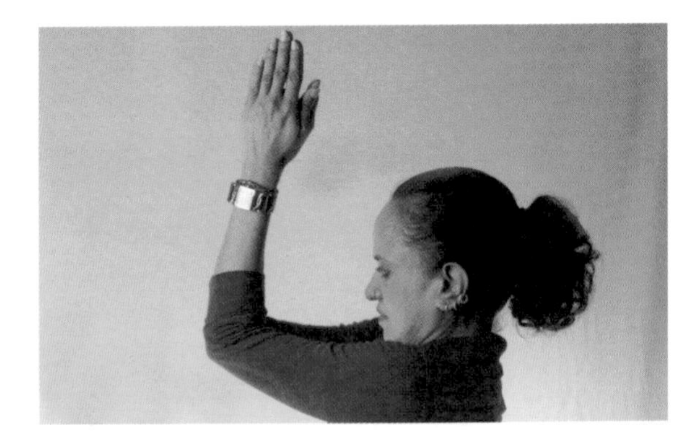

How it works

- Opens up the shoulders, working that joint.
- Powers entire arms, so they can relieve some pressure off the shoulder.
- Tones and strengthens the entire upper torso.

Other benefits

- Opens up the lungs.
- This in turn elevates one's mood.
- Increases mental alertness.

PRANAMASANA (PRAYER POSE, ADVANCED VERSION)

Method

- May be done seated or standing.
- Place hands together as above, palms touching.
- The arms must touch from fingers, right down to the elbows.
- Inhale, raise elbows to face-level.
- Exhaling, lower arms, curving spine a bit to place elbows at belly.

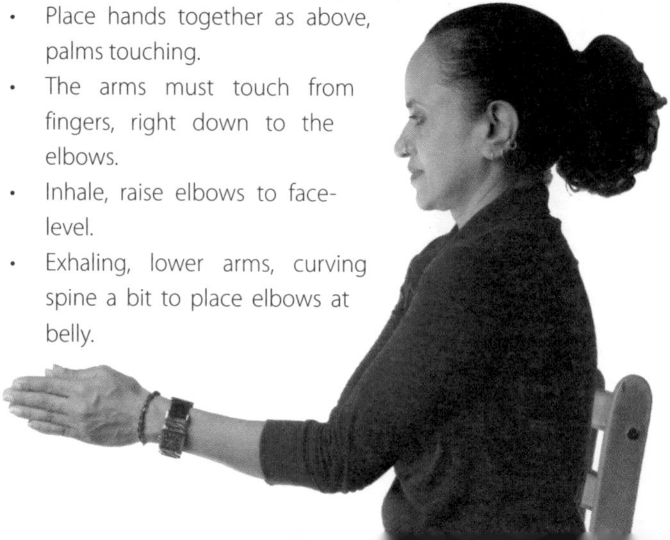

- Inhale. Exhaling, lower the hands further, with elbows still at the stomach to extend the stretch.
- Hold on for a few seconds, breathing normally.
- Release.
- Repeat three to five times.

How it works

Same as above, more enhanced.

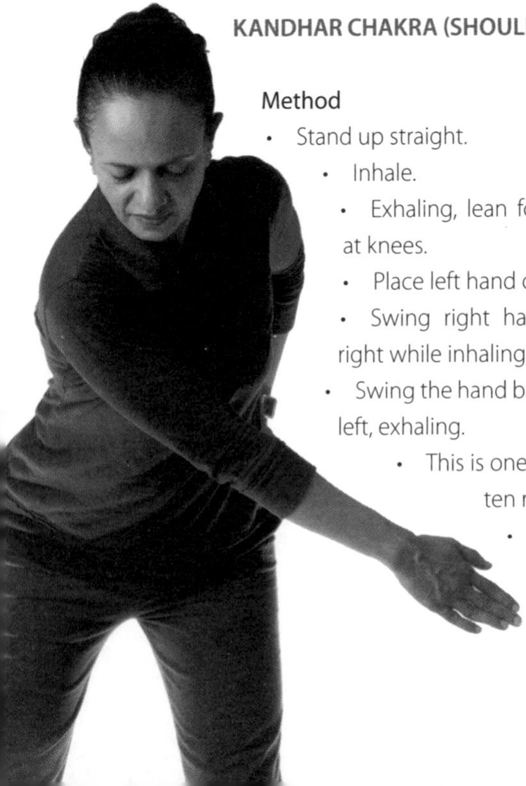

KANDHAR CHAKRA (SHOULDER CIRCLE)

Method

- Stand up straight.
- Inhale.
- Exhaling, lean forward, bending at knees.
- Place left hand on left hip.
- Swing right hand from left to right while inhaling.
- Swing the hand back, from right to left, exhaling.
- This is one round. Do up to ten rounds.
- Switch hands to swing left hand in a similar fashion.

How it works

- It lubricates the shoulder joint.
- Works out the large shoulder muscles.
- It works on the supporting neck muscles.

Other benefits

- When done with breath awareness, this exercise induces mental focus.
- Prevents frozen shoulder and neck pain.
- It works on immunity-strengthening acupressure-points on the back.

What else?

- All these exercises also prevent and **heal neck problems**.
- Since neck muscles and upper back muscles also support muscles used for respiration, they **boost lung capacity**.
- Since enhanced breathing keeps us upbeat, these moves also positively affect the mind, keeping us **mentally stimulated**.

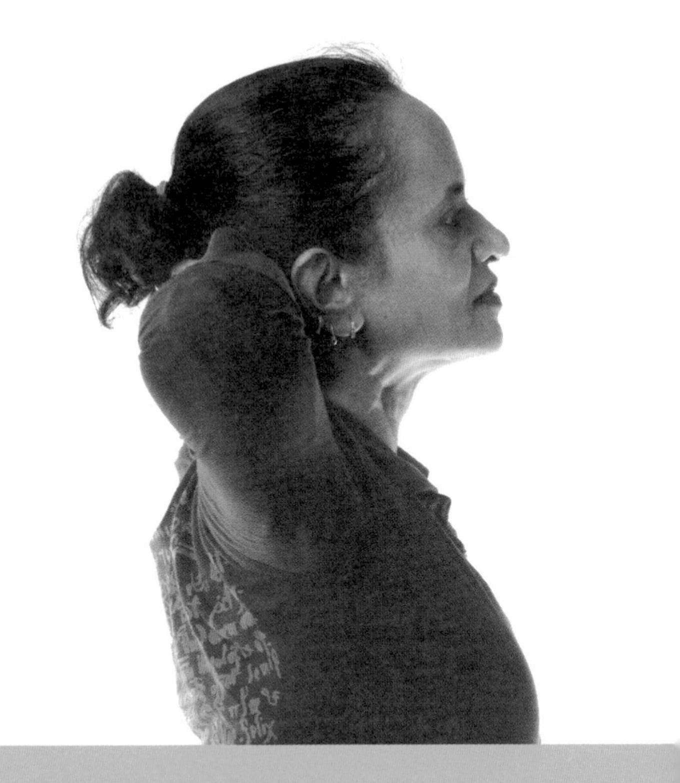

ZAP CHRONIC FATIGUE

A fast-paced, ambitious, driven lifestyle, combined with erratic food and sleep habits, can spark off a new age problem now accorded an official name — chronic fatigue syndrome.

A dislike for crowded places, which can result from commuting in congested public transport; a fear of intimidating bosses or office bullies on the prowl; or even an alteration in habits or daily routine, can spark this syndrome. Surprisingly, the last could include what are normally seen as welcome or happy events in one's life, like a wedding, holidays, a new addition to the family, a promotion, even a shift in residence or any major family event!

Earlier dismissed clinically as just something 'in the head', doctors have now started catching on to the warning signs of this syndrome. This is because CFS has actual physical symptoms which could be dangerous to ignore — low blood pressure or high blood pressure, anaemia, low-intensity but chronic fever, weight loss or weight gain, muscle loss, loss of appetite, headache, insomnia, sleep apnea, thyroid malfunction, heart ailments. The emotional symptoms include low motivation or disinterest in regular activity, chronic depression, failing memory, indecisiveness, panic attacks or lethargy. This swathe of symptoms, sometimes surfacing individually or targeting you with multi-pronged viciousness, can confound doctors too. Also, whether CFS creates these symptoms or is caused by these triggers, is not clear. Adding to this confusing scenario are other contributors, like bad ergonomy; new-age gadgets with their radiations, the effects of which are yet to be studied in depth; ill-maintained office spaces or air-conditioning; continuous exposure to artificial lighting; even proximity to some office gadgets like scanners or photocopying machines can be the physical causes for CFS.

Having a short but sensible set of yogic exercises which can build your stamina, up your immunity and elevate the mood will armour you against this Hydra-headed problem. We have for you some classic poses that are powerfully therapeutic; some are used to relieve emotional blockages (like the eagle pose), while the classic cat and energy-release (pawan muktasana) are cure-all exercises that release you from physical maladies ranging from migraine to spinal stiffness. Their simplicity disguises the miraculous impact they have. They have been specifically chosen for their potency, since a problem like CFS creeps into your life insidiously.

GARUDASANA (EAGLE POSE)

Method

- May be done seated or standing.
- Inhale.
- Cross hands at chest, passing right arm over the left one.
- Weave the hands, passing left hand over right wrist, thus interlocking fingers as shown in the picture.
- Exhaling, lift the entwined hands so elbows are now at face-level. After a few weeks of practice, when flexibility has been gained, you may gently touch your nose with the hands.
- Hold on for a few seconds, breathing evenly.
- Then, inhaling, drop hands back to chest level.

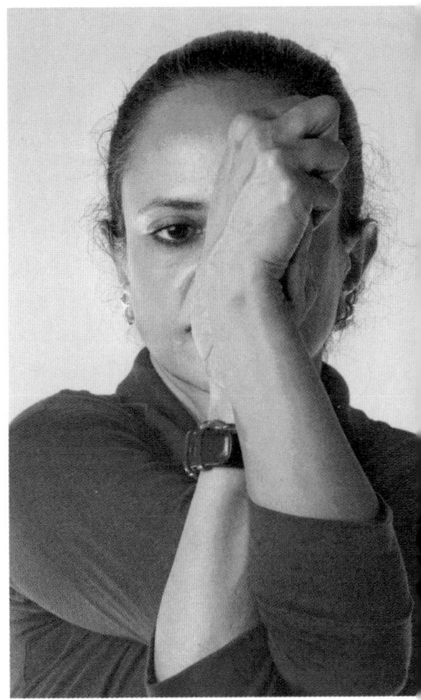

- Exhale, raise hands again, so they are face level.
- Repeat a few times.
- Relax and bring arms back to the starting position. Release the interlocked fingers. Rest.
- Then cross right arm over the left, to repeat the sequence.

Points to note

The posture, called the 'classic eagle pose', is a real stamina builder. This original version can be ranked as an intermediate pose. You can do it after perfecting the upper limb workout, as instructed before. The original version enhances mental stamina and limb coordination.

How it works

- Releases stiffness of shoulders. This can bring about stress relief.
- Opens the chest, to boost respiration.
- Works on the immune gland.
- Harmonises both sides of the brain, making you centred.

Other benefits

- Prevents neck pain.
- Helps with computer-related problems like Repetitive Strain Injury (RIS).
- Shapes and tones entire arms.
- Is therapeutic for middle- and upper-spinal problems.

GARUDASANA (EAGLE POSE, ADVANCED VERSION)

Method

- Cross hands at chest, passing right hand over left, interlocking fingers while inhaling.
- Exhaling, lift elbows higher than in the previous posture.
- Elbows must be almost at face level, while hands pass over the head.
- Continue breathing, holding the pose. Do it a few times.
- Release, repeat with left hand passing over right.

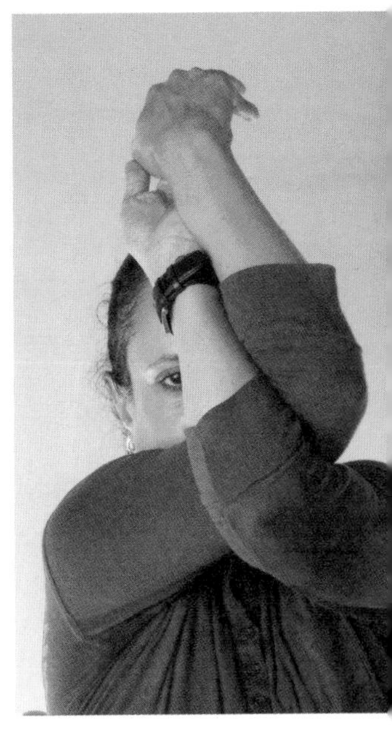

Points to note

This is a powerful stretch. Advance to this exercise only after practising the first version for several weeks.

How it works

- Same as above, more enhanced.

Other benefits

- It also boosts respiration, opens the chest, decongesting lungs.
- It is mood uplifting.

PAWAN MUKTASANA (ENERGY RELEASE POSE)

Method

- Stand up straight. (This version is done standing. Another version, seated, is presented later in the book. This one involves your sense of balance too.)
- Inhale. Bend right leg at knee.
- Exhale, lift right knee as high as you can.
- Inhale. Exhaling, hug knee to your body — either at belly or at chest, depending on your flexibility.
- Hold, breathing normally.
- Release. Repeat a few times.
- Repeat for the other side.

Points to note

All yoga schools unanimously agree that the power of this posture lies in its ability to unlock blocked nadis or energy channels in the body.

How it works

- Tones liver.
- Prevents acidity.
- Is an energising exercise.
- Gives a gentle, complete traction to spine.
- Provides a powerful leg stretch.

Other benefits

- Is a cure-all pose, used as the safest therapeutic practice in all ailments, ranging from high blood pressure, cardiac trouble, migraine, digestive woes, spinal stiffness and diabetes.

MARJARI ASANA (CAT STRETCH)

Method

- Stand up straight.
- Inhale deeply.
- Exhaling, curve the abdomen in with force so that the spine also curves. Hold the pose for a few seconds.
- You may continue breathing normally. Or, if not suffering from any cardiac ailment or high blood pressure, hold your breath for four seconds.
- Release. Repeat thrice.

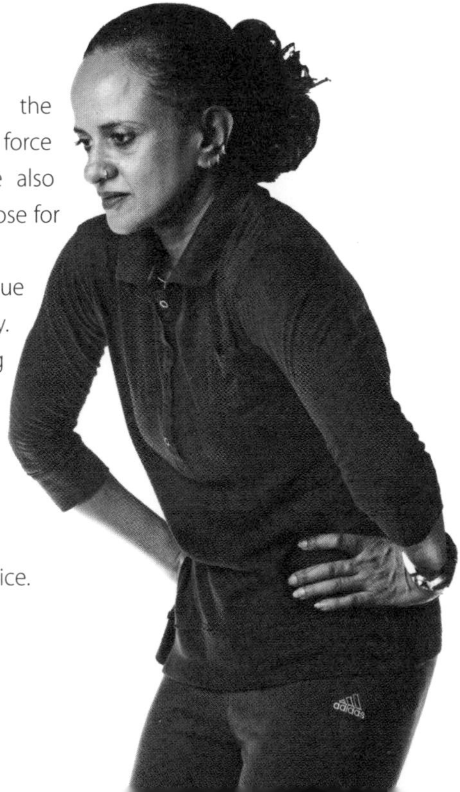

Points to note

This is one of the rare yoga poses that is absolutely safe for women to perform during menstruation. It may be ranked amongst the no-contraindication poses in yoga.

How it works

- Is a cure-all pose.
- Is used to treat migraine.
- The caved-in abdomen applies powerful pressure on the uro-genital system, helping treat ailments here.
- Is used to tackle pre-menstrual syndrome and menstrual cramps.
- Helps control acidity and digestive problems.
- Arching the back relieves spinal stiffness.
- The expansion and release of the torso works out the respiratory system by powering the supporting muscles, boosting breath capacity.

Other benefits

- This is regarded as an anti-ageing exercise.
- Tones, trims legs.

PAWAN MUKTASANA (ENERGY RELEASE POSE)

Method

- May be done seated or standing.
- Place hands behind head or neck, interlocking fingers. An ideal and comfortable spot is the base of the skull.
- Elbows are held out, pointed outwards.
- Inhale. Exhaling, bring elbows together in front of the face as if to touch one with the other (but that will not be possible, just bring the elbows as close as possible).
- Inhale, open elbows out.
- This is one round.
- Do five to ten rounds.

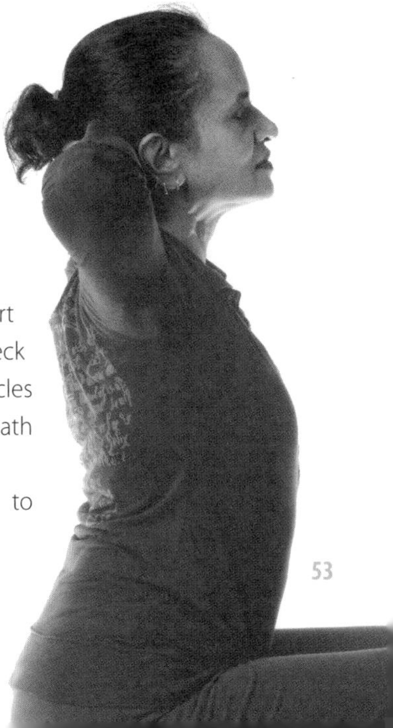

How it works

- It loosens the upper body, usually contracted with tension or a posture maintained for a long time.
- The muscles that support respiration, such as the neck muscles and shoulder muscles are relaxed, enhancing breath capacity.
- Chest muscles are flared to boost lung capacity.

Other benefits

- Enhanced breathing boosts one's mood.
- Breath sequencing enhances mental focus.

What else?

- These are **detox poses** which prime the liver and release it from lethargy.
- They are also **weight-loss aids**, because they improve metabolism and tone muscles.
- All lengthen the spine, powering the spinal nerves and **preventing postural defects**.
- All poses also help in **de-stressing**.
- They clear blocked energy channels, and provide a **quick pick-me-up**.

Cameron Diaz, as the svelte Charlie's Angel, introduced something called 'cobra yoga'. Gywneth Paltrow, on the other hand, practised the rigorous ashtanga yoga to lose pregnancy pounds. Madonna has stumped age and fat through the same genre of yoga. Lanky Christy Turlington published a book listing weight-loss amongst yoga's many benefits. Super singer Sting punctuated his India visit with interviews on his fascination for ashtanga yoga, while Hollywood heartthrobs Richard Gere and Tobey Maguire attribute their muscular litheness to yoga. Closer home, our desi Jane Fonda, Shilpa Shetty, has released a successful yoga DVD, and the gorgeous Kareena Kapoor, actor Rahul Bose and cricketer Rahul Dravid are self-confessed yoga enthusiasts.

Now, let's find out why yoga is favoured by the glitzy set.

FIGHTING FAT

- Because its effects are long-term.
- Though yoga's fat-busting effects may take a month's time to show up, it offers insurance against the yo-yo effects of other quicker fat-losing methods.

- Yoga exercises reach deep down to control glands and hormones responsible for hunger and satiety.
- New-fangled diet programmes may help in weight-loss, but also make the skin loose (since the underlying fat that provided elasticity has been lost), thus making people looked old and haggard. Yoga, on the other hand, helps in firming up the skin.
- Weight-loss in yoga is accompanied by building and toning of muscles. This ensures that you are losing weight even while not doing anything, since muscle has higher calorific needs than fat and greater metabolic burn .

Below are a few simple yogic fat-busters you can practise while at work.

SURYA MUDRA (HAND GESTURE)

Method

- Sit in meditative position.
- Shut your eyes.
- Press your ring finger down with the thumb.
- Do this with both hands.
- Hold for three to five minutes, repeat several times during the day.

Points to note

People with high blood pressure, heart problems, fever or inflammatory conditions should avoid this mudra since it increases body heat. It is ideal in a cold climate. It is also an ideal mudra while meditating or practising pranayama.

How it works

- It employs the homunculus-neurological map in human brain.
- It uses the Ayurvedic principle of elements in our body, and suppresses the earth element, which causes weight gain and/or difficulty in losing weight. It is used to control the kapha/water element in the body.
- Even a few minutes in this mudra will show that the body heat or metabolic fire goes up, as body temperature shoots up. This indicates the powerful impact of this posture.
- It is actively used to lose weight.

Other benefits

- Is used in treating and controlling diabetes.
- May be used in extreme cold conditions to heat up the body naturally.
- It may be used to relieve congestion.
- Also used in therapy for hypothyroidism.
- Relieves constipation.

UDDIYANA BANDHA (STOMACH LOCK)

Methods

- Place your hands on your waist.
- Inhale and exhale deeply a few times.
- Inhale. Exhaling forcefully, lock in the stomach muscles, caving in the spine.
- Hold the breath and lock for a few seconds.
- Relax stomach.
- Exhale lightly, before inhaling deeply.

Points to note

This exercise is also good for inflammatory problems of the gut, like ulcers, irritable bowel syndrome, hernia, heart ailments, blood pressure.

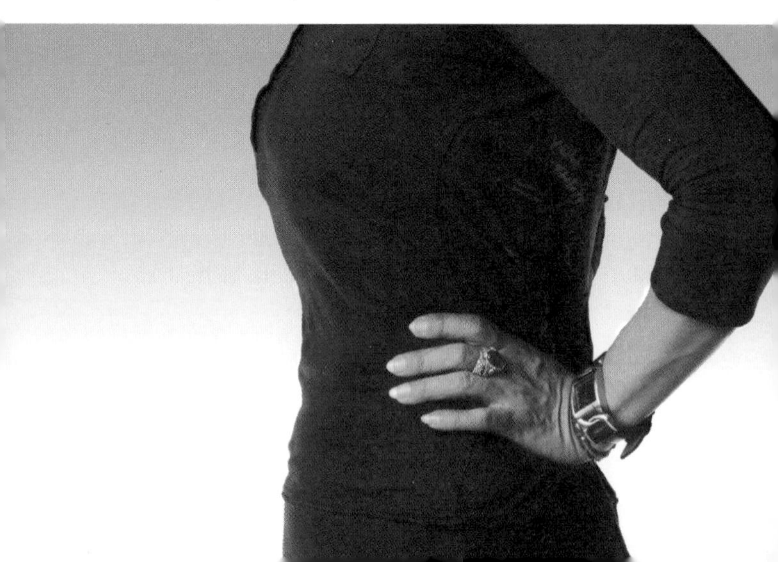

How it works

- It strengthens the gut, usually abused with wrong eating habits.
- It spikes metabolism. An abused gut becomes lethargic, and a falling metabolic rate leads to weight gain and malabsorption that in turn gives out wrong hunger signals.
- It prevents or controls digestive problems, which form the crux of obesity therapy.
- Relieves constipation.
- Is used to eject intestinal worms. Intestinal pests are often the cause behind wrong hunger signals. They also create a chronic nutrient deficiency, which in turn sparks hunger pangs.
- Builds willpower and mental stamina, thus powering our ability to have control over addictions.

Other benefits

- It reduces abdominal sagging.
- Is an anti-ageing practice.
- Is a stimulating practice, which spikes mental focus.
- If breath retention is practised and the duration of the final hold is increased progressively, willpower improves.

JANU NAMAN (KNEE PRESS)

Method

- Sit on a chair.
- Press feet on the ground. Inhale.
- Place hands on inner sides of the knees. Exhale.
- Inhaling, press both knees outwards and away from each other with your hands.
- Simultaneously, push your legs inwards, to create a resistance between the hands and legs.
- Hold this resistance as long as is possible, breathing normally throughout.
- Release. Repeat a few times.

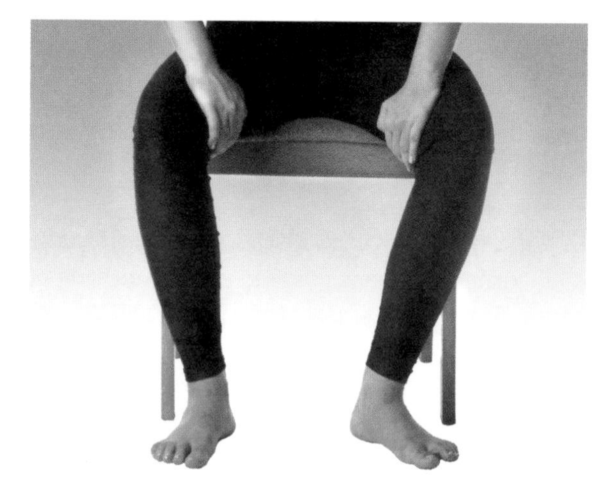

How it works

- All exercises that make the body work out or exert itself help fight fat.

Other benefits

- This works out the wrists and legs powerfully, using your own body for resistance training.
- Tones body, building muscle throughout.
- Improves stamina.

PADASANA (LEG POSE)

Method

- Stand in front of a chair, with enough distance to place the right heel on it, as shown below.

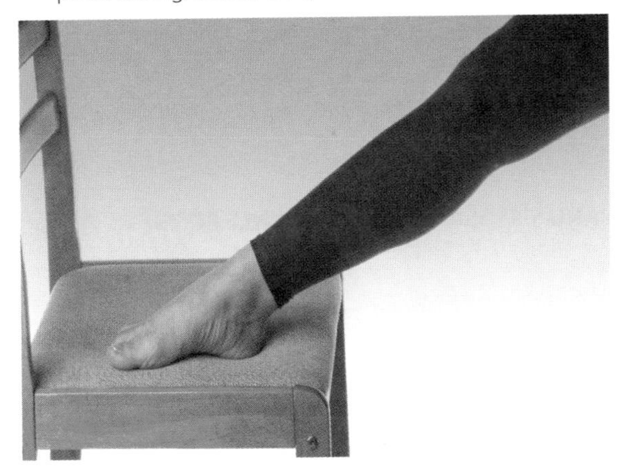

- The leg should be as straight as possible. Inhale.
- Flex toes towards your body. Then extend it away from the body with an exhalation.
- Do this a few times, with breath awareness.
- Repeat for the other leg.

Points to note

- Ensure that the leg on the chair remains straight. Most people slacken at the knee. This will reduce the impact.

How it works

As with the previous exercise.

Other benefits

- Strengthens, tones the entire leg.
- Powers the knee, preventing and helping control knee problems.
- This posture, done with breath awareness, boosts mental focus.

JANU SIRSASANA (HEAD-TO-KNEE POSE)

Method

- Place your heels on a chair as shown in the picture alongside.
- Inhale. Exhaling, bend your head towards the right knee.

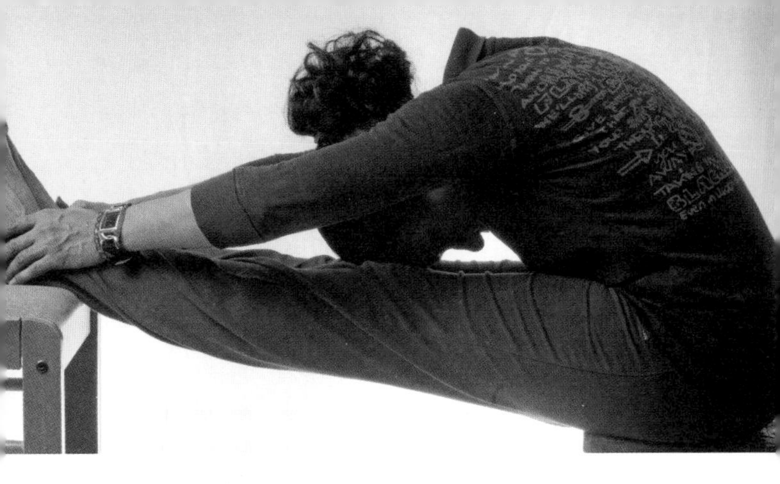

- Try to hold your toes. If that is difficult, hold the leg where you can.
- Continue breathing evenly. Release.
- Repeat a few times.
- Rest. Then repeat for the other leg.

Points to note

- With regular practice, and as the back becomes more supple, you can try to deepen the pose by moving your head closer to the knee.
- Those with a lower-back problem shouldn't bend too low.

How it works

- Powers digestion, increases metabolism, aids weight loss.
- Removes lethargy.

- Is therapeutic in diabetes, which is linked to weight gain.

Other benefits

- Is a cure-all pose, used in most ailments of the body and mind.
- Prevents spinal problems, especially upper-back ones.
- Is amongst the few poses used in treating knee problems.

What else?

- These resistance training exercises, adapted as chair yoga, **help tone and work out the entire leg.** Strong legs rectify and remove postural defects by taking the load off the spine. This prevents later lifestyle problems such as chronic knee ache and lower back pain. Along the way, these poses also shape the legs.
- Most weight-loss postures are also linked to building **mental stamina and focus**, since the ability to control diet is largely tied to this.
- These exercises are also **anti-ageing,** since obesity can damage inner organ systems drastically, ageing them.
- Most poses are also **cure-all poses,** since the obese also suffer from other problems, caused by hormonal imbalances that the fat unleashes inside the body.

It is rather unfortunate that people who are required to be up and about on their legs most of the time, because of their jobs or household chores, end up having weaker lower limbs. This sets off other unrelated, often misdiagnosed problems concerning the nervous system, the circulatory system, and the master organ — the heart.

Even the drugs consumed, as a short-term relief method, cannibalise vital nutrients which in turn weaken the body by depleting magnesium, needed for tissue health and repair. This further weakens the powerful leg muscles needed to keep the entire body upright. Undiagnosed diabetes (also related to magnesium malabsorption or deficiency) is also related to leg problems, including night-time cramps.

LEG TONE-UP

Lower spine problems and the health of one's legs are also related. Stiff legs (caused by misguided exercises like treadmills, running without warm-ups or stretches, or playing sports that favour one side over the other) are linked to an over-stiff spine. This can trigger problems anywhere along the spine, from the upper back right down to the lower parts. Acute knee problems are also caused when the large thigh or calf muscles are not supple enough to give the body adequate shock-absorbing capacity, thus burdening the delicate knees severely.

Anxiety has also been found to cause trembling in the leg. Mental fogginess may be caused by sitting in one place for a long time, because movement is essential to push blood to all parts of the body, including to the brain. Blood movement is, as it is, restricted by gravity — our passive lifestyle only makes it even more difficult for the circulatory system. Weak legs translate into weak arteries. This compromises the heart's health, since this organ must now try harder to push the blood around. It is a given that those who have weak legs invariably also suffer from breathlessness even after casual, simple chores. This proves that oxygen transport is also affected.

The main villain in all this is an inactive lifestyle. But the next villain is the lack of a structured exercise programme in our lives. Doing these powerful leg stretches will open up your hips and work your legs. Most importantly, they will power your working day.

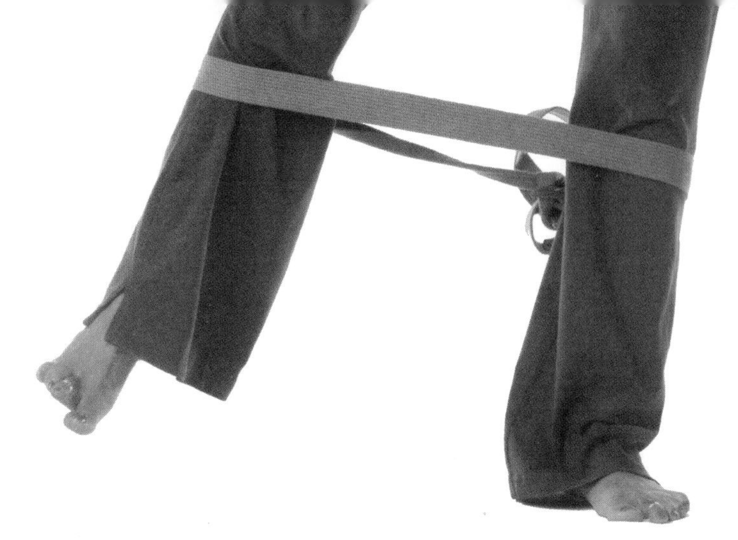

UTTHITA PADASANA (RAISED LEG POSE, BAND VERSION)

Method

- Have a band or belt or scarf ready.
- Tie ends, to make a loop that is about one foot long.
- Place the loop around the ankles or calves by stepping into the loop.
- Stand up straight. Hold on to a chair or table for support.
- Raise right leg up, sideways, towards the right, with an inhalation.
- Use the loop to create a strong resistance.
- Continue normal breathing, holding this pose for as long as possible.
- Release foot back to ground with an exhalation.

- Repeat three to five times.
- Relax, then repeat for the left leg.

How it works

- The resistance creates a powerful workout for the entire leg. Trims, shapes and tones lower limbs.
- The hip, and all major muscles, including that of the thigh and calf, are worked out.
- Prevents knee ache by strengthening the joint.

Other benefits

- Perks up the mind, improves concentration.
- Harmonises both sides of the brain, creating inner balance and emotional intelligence.
- Prevents hip fractures.
- Assures fat loss and muscular tone when number of repetitions is increased.

UTTHITA PADASANA (RAISED LEG POSE)

Method

- Stand up straight, with a chair or table for support, inhale.
- Exhaling, bend right leg at knee, and hold right ankle in your right hand.
- Inhale, lift bent leg sideways, towards your right.
- Initially raise only a few inches.

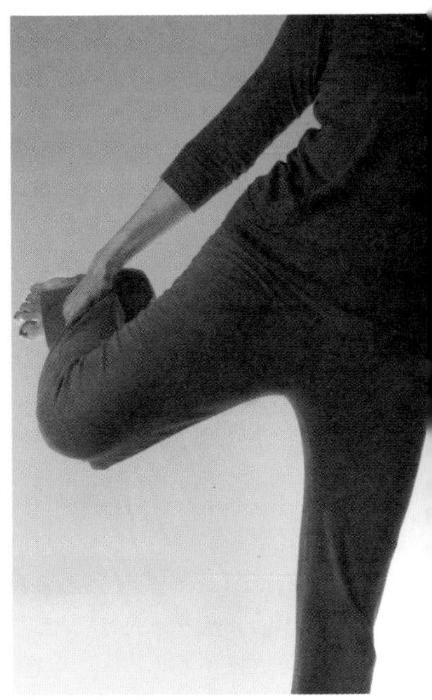

- Later, with regular practice, you may raise the leg higher, so your calf is parallel to the floor.
- Hold, breathing normally. Release, to return to starting pose. Rest foot back on the ground. Repeat a few times.
- Then repeat equal number of times for the other side.

How it works

Same as above.

Other benefits

- Opens up the hips.
- Offers relief in uro-genital problems.
- Enhances mood.

UTTAN PADASANA (LEG STRETCH POSE)

Method

- Stand up straight.
- Inhale to move right foot some distance away from the left.

- Point right foot out, towards the right. This takes pressure off the knee. The left foot may remain pointed forward.
- Exhale, squat lightly at the right knee.
- Hold for a few seconds, breathing normally.

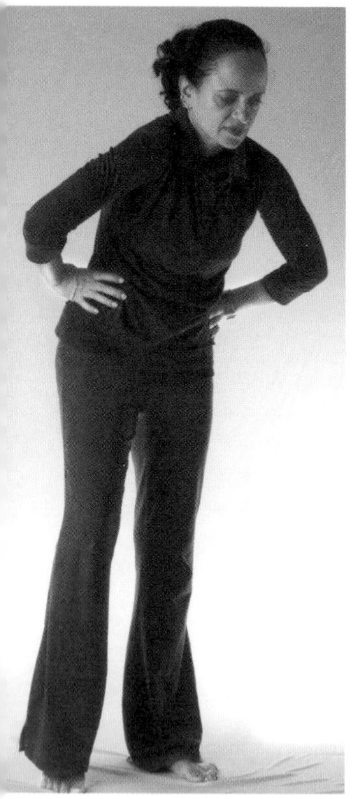

- Release, to return to starting pose.
- Repeat a few times.
- Rest, repeat for the other side.

Points to note

Avoid if you have severe knee pain.

How it works

- Shapes and tones the leg.

Other benefits

- Also builds mental stamina.
- It is demanding and challenging, thus encouraging fat burn.

UTKATASANA (SQUAT POSE, ADVANCED VERSION)

Method

- Stand up straight.
- Keep feet a foot apart. Feet remain pointing straight ahead. Inhale.
- Exhaling, squat deeply at both knees, so the body dips down.
- Hold the squat, breathing normally.
- Release, return to starting pose.
- Repeat a few times.

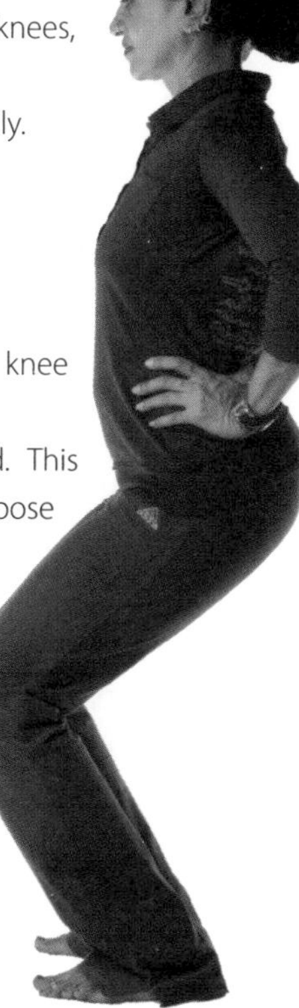

Points to note

- Avoid if you have severe knee problems.
- Avoid tilting the torso forward. This error reduces the impact of the pose substantially.

Benefits

As in the last asana, but more enhanced.

KAPOTASANA (PIGEON POSE)

Method

- Has to be done seated on a chair.
- Sit on the edge of the chair.
- Cross legs, passing right leg over left. Inhale.
- Exhaling, press right foot down so that toes point towards the floor.
- If you are tall, it is likely your foot will touch the floor. Otherwise, just point it floorwards.
- Hold, breathing evenly, and then release. Do it a few times.
- Release. Cross left leg over right and repeat exercise equal number of times.

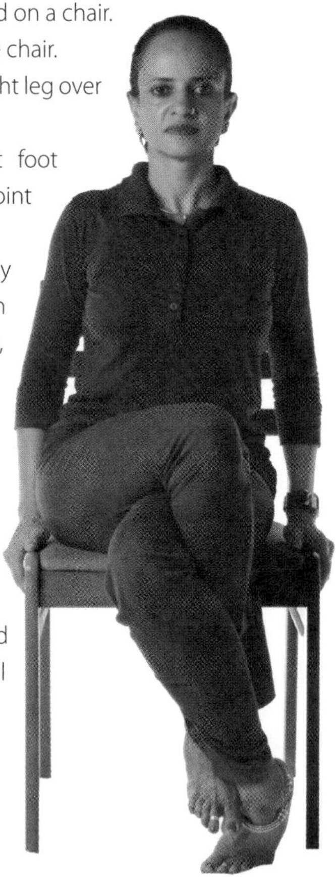

How it works

- Tones, shapes legs, especially calf

muscles.
- Improves posture by removing postural imbalances.

Other benefits

- Harmonises both brain hemispheres.
- Is calming, encourages mental focus.

What else?

- A sedentary lifestyle hits legs the worst. And even those who walk or stand for long periods (like stewards, airhostesses, receptionists, nurses, doctors) can have very stiff legs due to overload. Yogic leg stretches help both extremes of under-use and over-use by helping **legs get more supple, elastic and become better load-bearers**. This impacts our posture marvellously, improving carriage and confidence.
- Since right and left sides are worked in all these exercises, both **brain hemispheres are harmonised, creating better dialogue between them, helping with problem-solving abilities and boosting emotional intelligence** in our reactions to stress.
- Bodily imbalances are also removed. We do not realise that by favouring one limb over the other we invite postural distortions and disharmony in the body. These poses **remove such physical imbalances.**
- As explained, leg work also boosts **mental energy** because of better blood flow to the brain.

Doctors these days prescribe some measure of movement even in cases of spinal injury to quicken healing. No wonder then that a normal spine in a chronic state of disuse suffers the 'stress' of neglect.

An inactive lifestyle makes the spine progressively stiff. It suffers from de-conditioning, meaning its normal range of movement becomes less, while muscles surrounding it also lose their casual mobility. Kinesthetic intelligence — a body's innate wisdom on movements — improves only with regular activity. Muscular weakness surrounding the spine also means less support to our body frame, further burdening it, causing postural adjustments that are actually defects. In fact, even abdominal sagging is common amongst those with a weak spine since the inactivity also means your stomach muscles have lost

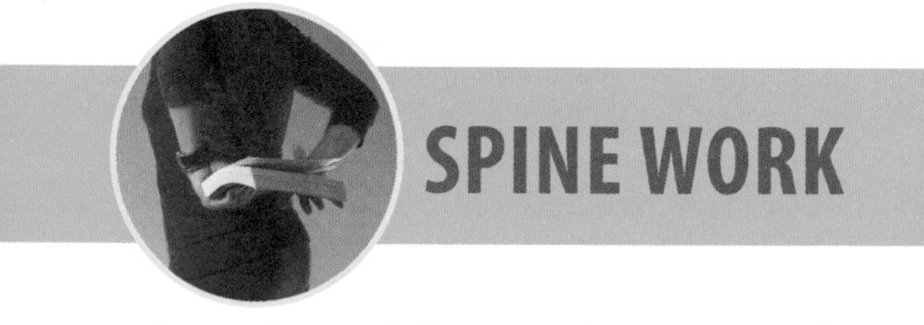

SPINE WORK

tone, and your spine's curvature becomes unnaturally deeper to accommodate this bulging belly.

Inactivity, it has been found, can seriously compromise your brain's control over the lower pelvic region. So, those dreaded stories of hip fractures amongst progressively younger generations is due to the fact that the brain's command over this region fails suddenly, causing the collapse from within.

To reduce swelling and inflammation in injured discs, rehab exercise in a progressive fashion is recommended because normal spinal health depends on motion for diffusion of fluids and nutrients in the spine. In a normal spine, the shock-absorbing cushioning disc between vertebrae can degenerate with prolonged inactivity, causing the spine to get stiffer and suffer greater shock each time you move. Popping pain-killers can only offer short-term relief and has serious side-effects.

Spinal problems are obviously not relegated just to your back. Upper back problems can cause debilitating headaches, vertigo and arm pain, including the excruciating frozen shoulder. Lower back pain, which requires the longest rehab treatment, can cause mood swings, severe leg pain, postural defect, knee pain (due to load on the delicate joint).

Use these the following exercises to prevent all such spinal mishaps.

UTTAN PADASANA (LEG STRETCH)

Method

- Stand up straight.
- Hold a chair or a table for support.
- Inhale, moving right foot about one foot away.
- Continue normal breathing, lifting the heel up and pointing your toe to the floor.
- If necessary move the right foot further, since tall people may need distance between feet to enhance the stretch.
- Feel the stretch extending from hip to tip of the toes.
- Relax back to starting position, to rest foot back on ground.
- Do a few times.
- Rest.
- Repeat for other side.

Points to note

Ensure you are not tilting forward or sideways. Keep the spine elongated and fully stretched for this pose to be effective.

How it works

- Strengthens and lengthens the spine.
- Firms and tones leg muscles, making them share the body's load more effectively.

Other benefits

- Increasing the number of repetitions can help build muscle tone and trim fat.
- Is a mood elevator, due to the improved circulation in the legs, which in turn boosts overall blood flow, particularly to the heart and the brain.

UDARKARSHANASANA (ABDOMINAL TWIST, WITH BOOK)

Method

- Keep a heavy book ready.
- Stand or sit on a chair.
- Inhale, lift the book with your right hand.
- Exhale, pass the book behind your back.

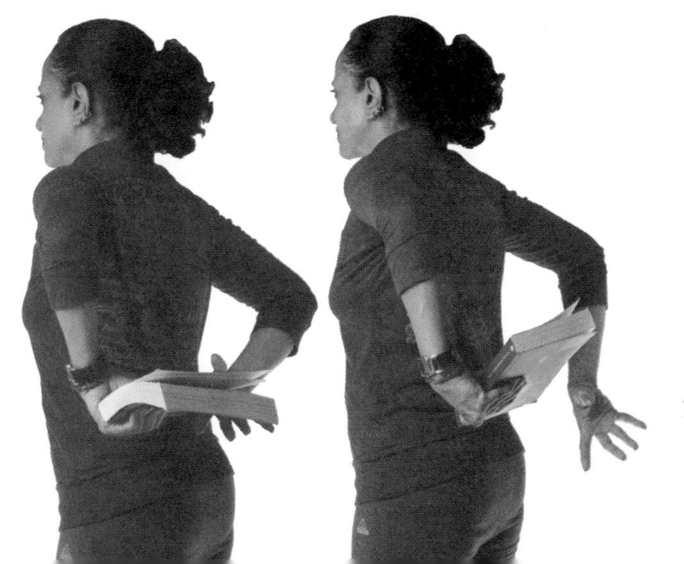

- Simultaneously reach for the book with your left hand and grasp it.
- Inhale, bringing the book forward. This completes one circle.
- Do five to ten times.

How it works

- Works shoulders, preventing neck-related problems, including frozen shoulder.
- Tones spinal nerves.

Other benefits

- Gives a gentle spinal workout.
- Works the digestive system, boosts metabolism.
- Improves hand, finger and brain coordination.
- Brings an element of fun due to the simple challenge involved, uplifting the mood.

TADASANA (PALM TREE POSE)

Method

- May be done seated or standing.
- Use a tie or a scarf or a dupatta for this exercise. It should be two feet or more in length.
- Hold the band with both hands, in front of you. Inhale, raising arms overhead, stretching the band as firmly as you can.

- Expand the stretch as much as you can. Arms should remain straight; ensure that you do not bend your elbows.
- Breathe normally in the posture, holding it for ten seconds or so.
- Release. Repeat a few times.

Points to note

If you have cardiac problems, hold the band in front of you instead of above your head.

How it works

- Provides a full body stretch, particularly at the upper torso.

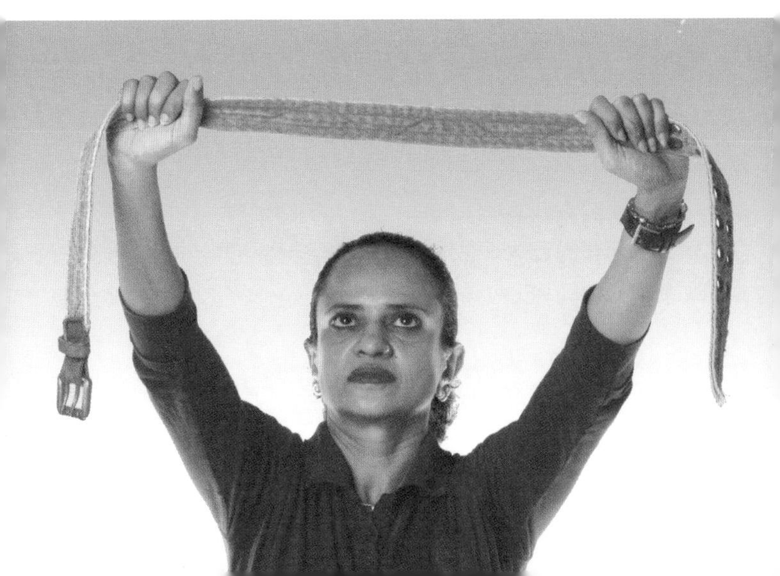

- Provides a spinal traction, a preventive in all spinal problems.

Other benefits

- Expands the rib cage, boosting respiration, which uplifts the mood.
- This is a cure-all pose, giving the whole body a good stretch and encouraging overall blood flow.

TADASANA (PALM-TREE POSE)

Method

- May be done seated or standing.
- Hold the band behind you.
- Inhale, raising and stretching the band behind you as much as you can.
- Hold this final pose, breathing normally. As in the previous exercise, ensure arms remain straight and do not bend at elbows.
- Release with an exhalation. Repeat a few times.

Points to note

Avoid in case you have cardiac problems, or do it in a phased manner.

Other benefits

- Same as above, more enhanced.
- Arms become toned.

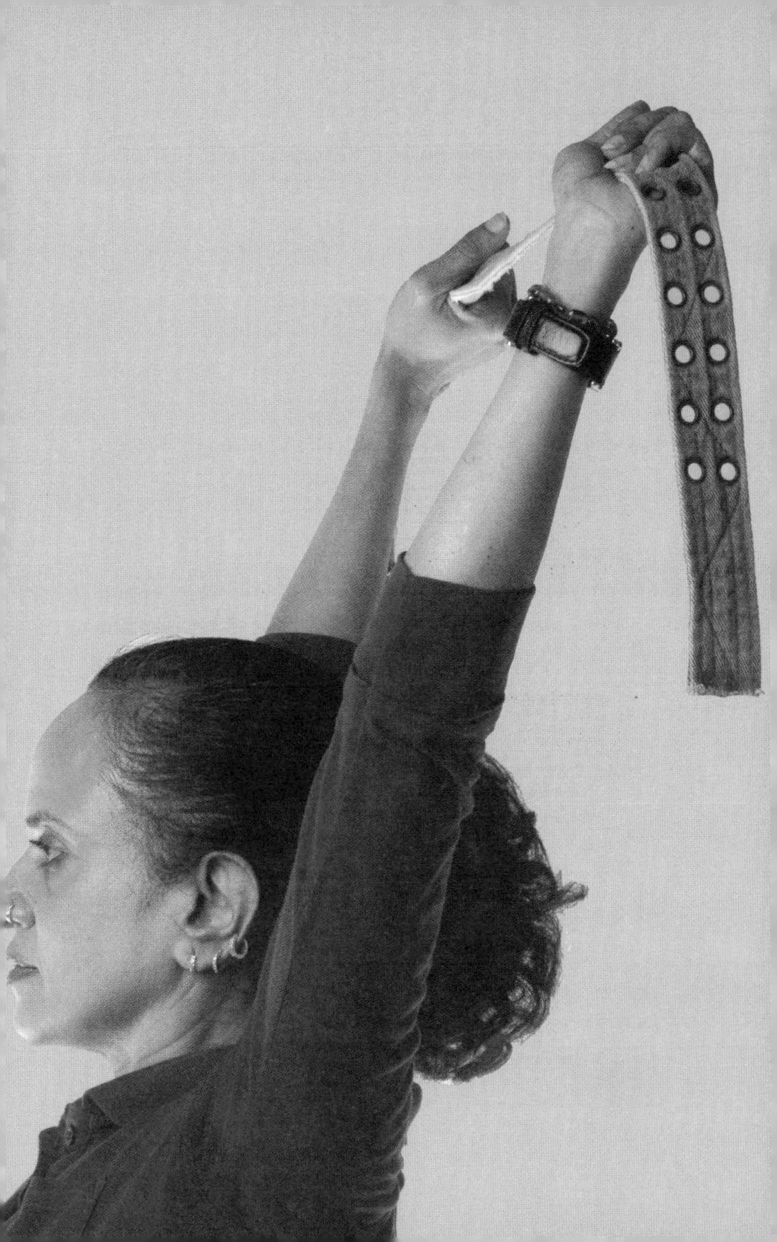

ARDHA CHANDRASANA (CRESCENT POSE, SEATED VERSION)

Method

- Sit up straight, on the edge of a chair.
- Inhale. Lift both hands above the head.
- Arch back, bending spine deeply, lifting head to look at hands.
- Hold for a few seconds, breathing normally. Relax to starting position.

Points to note

- If you have space and are not inhibited about practising these exercises, try these poses standing. They are powerful poses which will not only keep you trim, but boost your mental and physical stamina.

How it works

- Works out the entire spine and even tones spinal nerves.

Other benefits

- Expands the chest, boosting respiration.
- Is an instant pick-me-up.
- Tones arms.
- Boosts metabolism and digestion to fight obesity.

What else

- Keeping the spine supple may help **prevent several ailments, like knee ache, back pain and obesity.** The health of the spine is related to the rest of the major systems that are near it, in the torso and the skull.
- Recent research has shown that **mental alertness and brain rejuvenation** are promoted by spinal exercise since the spinal nerves are toned.
- A weak spine can negatively affect moods, through physical causes like weakened breathing. Both are taken care of by these exercises, which **boost lung volume and uplifts the mood**.
- **Body aesthetics is taken care of** in all spinal exercises — better carriage, greater confidence, better voice modulation, and therefore enhanced communication and self-presentation, all depend on a youthful spine.
- Spinal weakness also means abdominal sagging, which is symptomatic of digestive weakness, including obesity and unexplained weight gain. These **exercises prevent such weight gain.**

DEFUSING ACIDITY

Today acidity has become such an accepted part of our lives that nobody really feels embarrassed discussing it, even though it triggers socially awkward symptoms like flatulence, belching, burping, retching and halitosis.

The causes of acidity — either hypoacidity (caused by food rotting in your gut) or hyperacidity (where there is so much acid that it causes inflammatory conditions in the gut) — can be easily associated with our modern-day lifestyles. Eating meals hastily (breakfasting on the go), or absentmindedly (spooning in business lunches, or munching during your favourite TV soap) also cause these problems. Excess food, erratic meals, skipping meals, excessive consumption of refined stuff like white rice, processed flour or white sugar have become staple. An overdose of bottled drinks, dependence on caffeine to kick-start the day, wrong food choices, routinely eating packaged or re-heated food, mixing foods indiscriminately since we have to make do with what is available while working — all these can severely affect the gut.

Another very relevant cause of acidity is a sedentary lifestyle. Remaining passive for long hours compromises the body's ability to dump toxic substances. A particularly noxious habit, is having an extended and long dinner which runs too close to our bed-time, and this is a major contributor to overall ill-health, particularly of the gut. Our body has its own bio-rhythm, and post-sunset the digestive system is already winding down. We wake it up and force-feed it, so it goes right back to sleep without doing its job. The food stuffed into the stomach then has no option but to rot, causing a real toxic environment there.

Anybody with a history of acidity is also aware that stress is a big culprit. An anxious or overwrought mind hits the digestive function acutely. Do the following yoga moves for instant and quick relief.

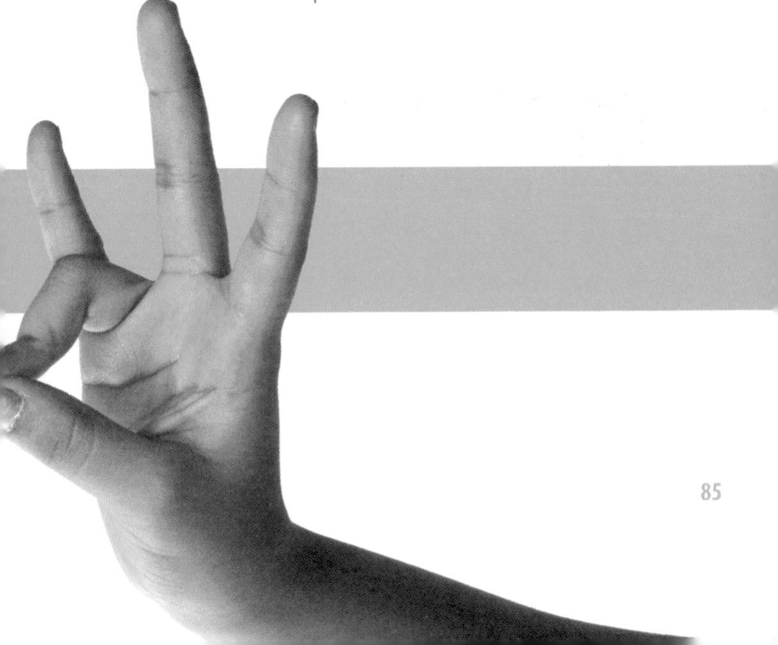

JAL SHAAMAK MUDRA (WATER-DECREASING HAND GESTURE)

Method

- Ideally done seated.
- Press little finger down with thumb. Do for both hands.
- Sit with closed eyes, with the hands on knees for a minimum of three minutes.
- May be done several times during the day in acute attacks.

Points to note

Mudras are like medicine. They may be used for specific problems and discontinued when the problem is under control.

How it works

In eastern therapies, the thumb is believed to represent the fire element and the little finger the water element. Pressing it down controls the excessive water (in this case acids). The thumb also experiences a pressure thus reducing the fire element or inflammatory conditions.

Other benefits

- It offers relief in congestion.
- It is soothing in diarrhoea.
- It is therapeutic in menorrhagia or excessive bleeding during menstruation.

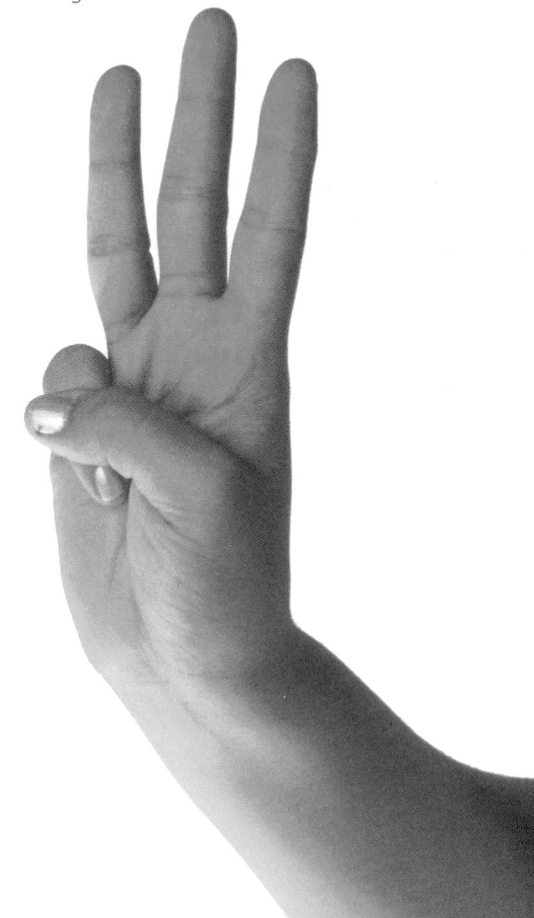

PRITHVI VARDHAK (EARTH-INCREASING HAND GESTURE)

Method

- Ideally done seated.
- Lightly press the tip of your ring finger with the tip of your thumb. Do so for both hands.
- Sit with closed eyes, with the back of the hands resting on your knees for a minimum of three minutes.
- May be done several times during the day in acute attacks.

How it works

As the name suggests, in ayurvedic parlance this increases the earth element and reduces the fire element.

Other benefits

- Improves energy levels.
- Removes excessive heat and dryness from the body.
- Relieves inflammatory conditions of the stomach, including hyperacidity.
- Soothing in heating conditions, as in fever.

PAWANMUKTASANA (ENERGY RELEASE POSE)

Method

- To be done seated on a chair.

- Inhale, bending right leg at knee, raising right foot to place it on the edge of a chair, near the hip, as shown.
- Exhale, passing both hands round the knee, to hug it closer to the body.
- Inhale and release the leg, placing it back on the floor.
- Do thrice.
- Repeat for the left leg.

How it works

- The pressure on the stomach soothes the gut and massages the entire digestive tract.
- The pressure also relieves and rejuvenates the stress glands.
- Encourages peristalsis and relieves flatulence.

Other benefits

- It is a cure-all pose, therapeutic in diabetes and high blood pressure.
- Is amongst the safest poses and is also one of the most healing poses.
- Opens the spine, and removes body stiffness.
- Prepares the body for more advanced poses.

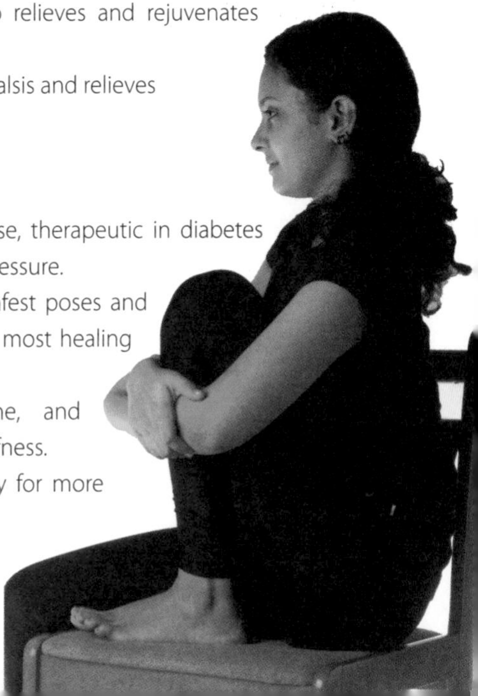

DWIPADA PAWANMUKTASANA (DOUBLE LEG ENERGY RELEASE POSE)

Method

- To be done seated in a chair.
- Inhale, bending both legs at knees.
- Simultaneously raise legs to place both feet at the edge of the chair, near hip, as shown in the picture below.
- Exhale, place both hands around bent knees, hugging them as close as possible to the body.
- Inhale, release legs, placing them back on the ground.
- Repeat a few times.

How it works and other benefits

Same as above, more enhanced.

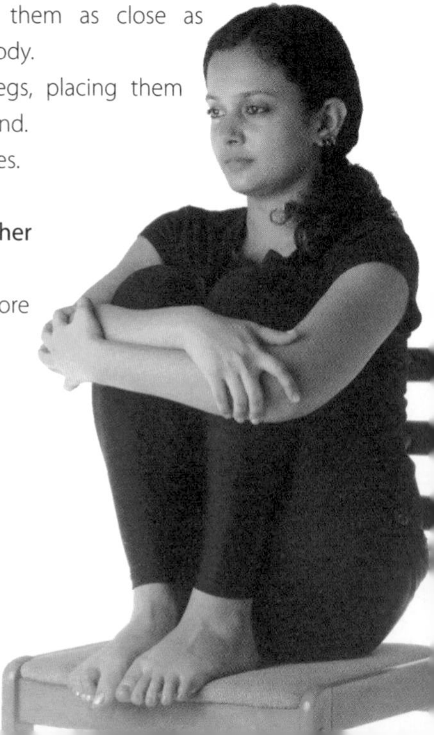

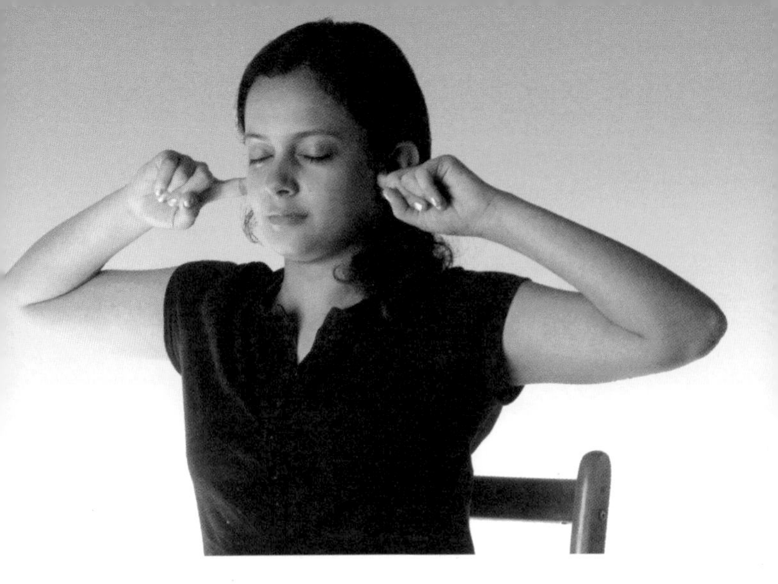

BHRAMARI (HUMMING BEE)

Method

- Sit up straight.
- Shut eyes.
- Place index finger of each hand on each ear (as shown in the picture above).
- Inhale, exhale consciously a few times.
- Inhale deeply.
- Begin to hum softly, feeling the 'mmm' vibrate in your face, throat, chest and abdomen.
- Extend the 'mmm' sound as long as you comfortably can.
- Relax. Keeping your eyes shut, repeat a few times.

Points to note

- The fingers in the ear enhance the hum. However, this may be dispensed with if practising in a public place.
- Avoid if feeling depressed or have ear infections.
- This pranayama (breathing practice) may be done several times during the day, particularly if you wish instant relief from stress.

How it works

- The humming sound is soothing, having a healing impact.
- It is a powerful de-stressing tool.
- The soft vibration has a vacuum-cleaner effect on all the sinuses on the cheeks and face, which affect the nitric oxide levels here. This positively impacts oxygen absorption.
- The lungs are emptied of their dregs of old air, impacting our moods and all our major systems.

Other benefits

- Is powerfully healing, used to treat all ailments.
- Calms one immediately.
- If the exhalation is long, it increases metabolism.
- Helps treat insomnia.
- Relieves anxiety, anger.

What else?

- All exercises that help relieve acidity also have a **de-stressing effect.** Since stress and acidity levels are linked, these poses are designed to relieve mental knots.
- Most exercises dealing with acidity are also **cure-all ones**, since acidity is both a symptom as well as the cause of various other ailments.

It is said that eighty per cent of our sensory distractions and information overload happen through our eyes. Add to this burden the new-age onslaught of gadgets and gizmos which compromise eye health even further.

When eyes strain to see, or are worked continuously, the mind interprets it as stress. This explains why we may feel extreme fatigue at the end of a long, chair-bound day mostly spent staring at a computer screen. Air-conditioning actually dehydrates our eyes. Again, since the movement of the eyes is restricted to a small area of focus, the natural suppleness of the muscles that hold the eyeballs is also compromised, causing vision problems, and red, gritty eyes. The latter happens because we forget to blink when movement of the eye muscles is restricted. It is said that we blink almost twenty to forty per cent

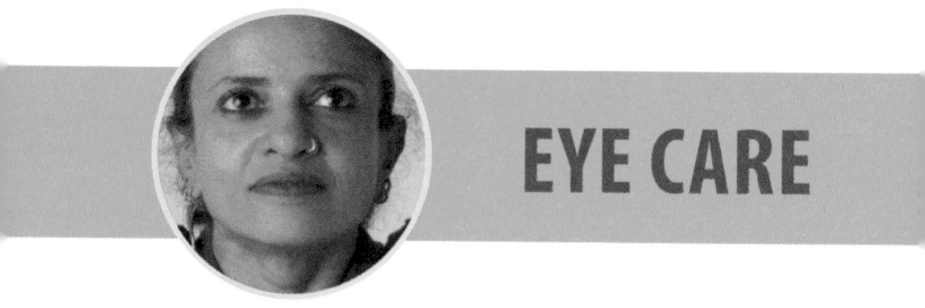

EYE CARE

less while doing such work. The eye's health depends on continuous and automatic blinking, since the film of moisture clears the eyes and the closure of the eyelids gives our eyes a short but much-needed rest.

Seeing that stress and vision are so intimately linked, it is clear that excessive mental tension will strain the eyes. Again, focusing intensely on anything also strains the eyes. The posture we assume while we focus and strain, contracting our neck muscles, also cramp the spine at those spots where the optic nerve passes, further hurting our vision. Vision affects posture, how we carry ourselves and may even contribute to subtle misalignment in our carriage that can, over time, hurt our backs, our knees and cause aches and pains far away from the cause.

Computer vision syndrome is now a recognised medical term, having reached the unfortunate epidemic status. Rest breaks, stretch breaks and yoga breaks are crucial to ensure that you can maximise your vision. Or contain the damage you have already inflicted on it.

'Palming' often can be a simple but effective relief not only to strained eyes, but also a stressed mind. To do this, rub your palms together gently, shut eyes and place the warm palms on your closed eyelids. Hold like this for a few minutes. If scrunched for time, try to hold for at least half a minute. Do this every few hours to rest and relieve over-worked eyes. Splashing water on the eyes immediately after a meal or after long hours of work can also refresh the eyes by encouraging a gush of blood to the face and eyes.

Staring steadily at any screen reduces natural moisture in the eyes, causing blurred vision, dry and red eyes, even glaucoma. It also denies the eyes of its constant, protective anti-bacterial wash. Staring can also cause wrinkles when you squint at the screen for long hours. These yogic eye exercises can prevent such job-related vision problems.

PRANAMASANA (PRAYER POSE)

Method

- May be done seated or standing.
- Place palms together in a namaste gesture.
- Fan out elbows as wide as you can.
- Place the hands so their base rests at the centre of your hairline.
- Inhale. Exhale deeply.
- Inhaling, tilt your head up gently. Look up.
- Ensure elbows remain fanned out.
- Hold this pose, breathing normally.
- Exhale. Release to return to starting point.
- Repeat a few times.

Points to note

The tilt is nominal, and must be gentle. Do not overexert the neck or the eyes while doing the exercises.

How it works

- It works out important acupressure points that fight ageing, including the sense organs.
- The upward tilt works the entire eye region, working subtle muscles around the eyes.

Other benefits

- This works out the entire neck region, removing ugly folds and sagging.

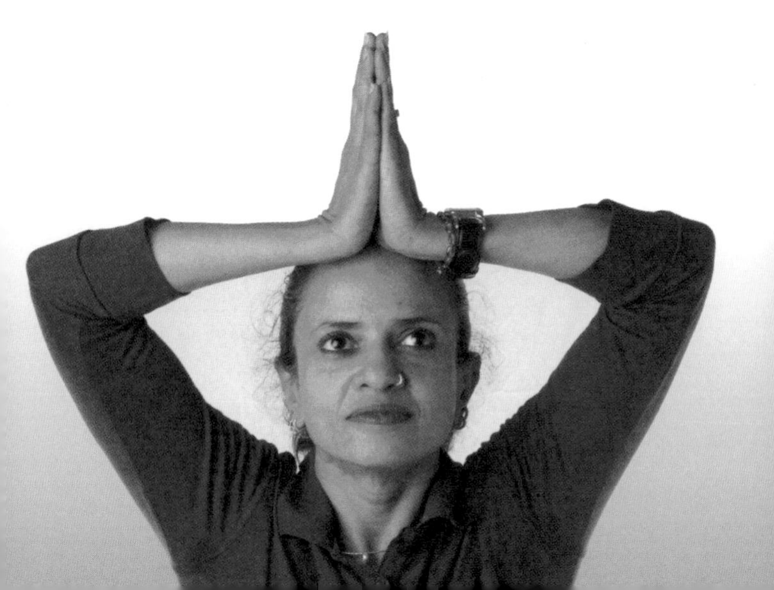

- It is a mood elevator, as are all upward facing poses.
- Such poses offer relief in respiratory ailments, since acu-points that relieve nasal congestion are activated.
- They sweeten the voice, adding power to voice delivery.
- Acu-points include Point 51 at the back of the neck (for lymphatic drainage or waste disposal).
- Others in the front of the neck and its base include those from 52 to 53, dealing with the voice box, facial skin tone and of the ear.
- Acu-points that help you maintain physical balance and the perfect posture are also tweaked.
- Points that balance the finicky thyroid gland needed for efficient metabolism are worked.

TRATAKA (YOGIC EYE EXERCISE, WITH BALL)

Method

- This may be done seated or standing.
- Ideal if you have a ball, but even a crumpled paper with something solid in it can be used as a substitute, as long as you can throw it with ease. You can also use your pen or any available object as a substitute.
- Throw the ball from right hand to the left in a curve.
- Blink once. Then throw ball from left to right hand.
- Do twenty-five times, each time blinking your eyes naturally in between each throw.

- Relax eyes at the end by palming: rub palms together, gently placing both palms on closed eyelids.
- Keep your eyes closed for half a minute or so before opening them to end the exercise.

How it works

- It re-trains you in the art of blinking. Blinking not only saves vision but also helps you read better by providing a minuscule but much-needed rest between words or sentences. 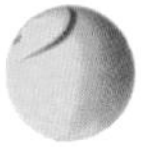
- This exercise improves peripheral vision, which is bound to degenerate with excessive staring at the computer screen.

Other benefits

- It also improves cognitive ability (ability to solve problems) through improved hand–brain coordination.

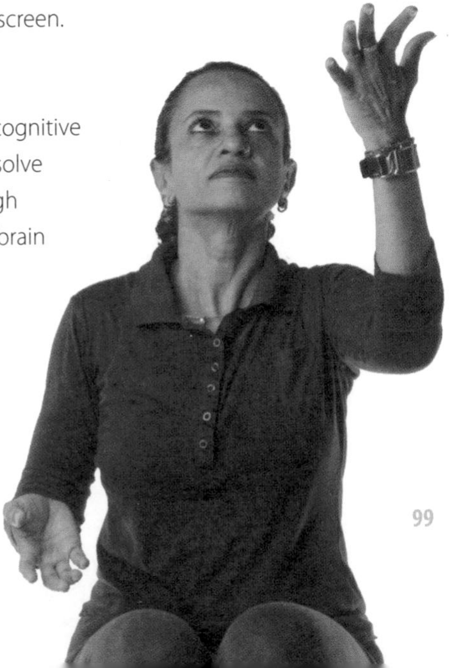

TRATAKA (YOGIC EYE EXERCISE, WITH PEN)

Method

- May be done seated or standing.
- This can be done with any linear object, like a pencil, your own thumb, etc.
- Hold object at eye-level, an arm's-length away from the face.
- Stare at the object.
- Then shift focus to tip of the nose.
- Relax, blinking naturally before repeating the exercises. Do ten to fifteen times.
- Relax eyes with palming, as described above.

How it works

- Improves telescopic vision of the eyes, plus retrains the eyes into adjusting to far–near movements.
- This corrects astigmatism. Also rectifies lazy eye syndrome (when one eye's vision is weaker than the other).

Other benefits

- Nose-tip gazing creates a deep, calming effect on the brain.

UTTANASANA (FORWARD-BENDING STRETCH POSE, RAG-DOLL VERSION)

Method

- Stand up straight.
- Inhale. Exhaling, reach out in front with both hands as if to touch the wall in front of you.
- Keeping lowering your upper body as you extend your exhalation.
- Now head should be facing thighs.
- Hands should hang loose.
- Stay in this relaxed, loose fashion, head hanging low for a while.
- Continue normal breathing throughout.
- To come up, inhale and slowly begin to raise your head and torso.
- The movement must be very slow and extremely relaxed. The slower you do this, the more relaxed you will feel.

Points to note

Avoid if you have lower backache.

How it works

- It relaxes the strained neck region, releasing the contraction that pinches spinal nerves, which in turn affects vision.
- It rushes blood to the face, including the eye region, which suffers less blood flow when we are inactive for long hours.

Other benefits

- Helps control diabetes.
- Is preventive and therapeutic in spinal problems.
- Aids weight loss.
- Keeps face young and smooth.
- Promotes mental calmness.
- Is therapeutic in anger.
- Helps control and relieve stress powerfully.

JAL MUDRA (HAND GESTURE OF WATER)

Method

- May be done seated or standing, but mudras are most effective when done meditatively.
- Touch the tip of your little finger with the tip of your thumb. Do it for both hands.
- Shut eyes, hold for three minutes at least for results.
- May be done several times during the day.

How it works

The mudra tweaks the homunculus man or the biological representation of the body parts in the brain, affecting important nerves associated with vision, physical hydration and mental calmness.

Benefits

- It hydrates the eyes.
- Is calming.
- Offers relief from excessive body heat, including fever.
- Relieves dryness of skin, eyes and hair.
- Relieves constipation.
- Is soothing in arthritic pain.

What else?

- Because of the relationship between the mind and our vision, keeping our eyes healthy may contribute tremendously towards **mental harmony**. These exercises are powerful de-stressers.
- Most of the eye exercises also work on subtle nerves and acu-points on the face that **control ageing.**

If you are prone to chronic headaches, one medical advice for you is to avoid sitting still for more than one hour at a stretch. Considering that we do this routinely, is it any wonder that headaches — in all their interesting variations from sharp to throbbing ones — have attained pandemic proportions?

Unlike most other ailments, a chronic headache becomes very difficult to diagnose. Also, there are an endless number of triggers, most of them lifestyle related. We can also safely add that some of these are psychosomatic, in that their origin has an emotional spark.

The following list of triggers should throw some light on this vague but nagging problem:

- Inactivity, which causes musculo-skeletal weakness that puts extra load on the spine, especially upper back.
- Muscle tension, also caused by the above reason. Often also caused by excessive stress.

- Eye-strain, again a job hazard these days.
- Inability to withstand natural light, again caused by remaining confined in artificial lighting for long hours or staring at computer/television screens for a long time.

- High blood pressure — caused by body stiffness that comes from an inactive or high-stress lifestyle.
- Poor working conditions — bad lighting; proximity to gadgets that release radiation or infra-red light (including photocopiers); poorly serviced air-conditioning; excessive crowding in office environs that create or mimic stress in the body; long hours of commuting.
- Spinal problems, including pinched nerves that arise from being seated in a slumped fashion for a long time.
- Stress itself is a major trigger.
- Allergic reactions, often released under stress when the body's auto-immune system turns upon itself.
- Respiratory ailments.
- Certain food types, often a hazard if you are routinely eating out.
- Erratic meal timings or skipped meals can cause a headache due to blood sugar swings.
- Erratic sleep timings is yet another trigger.
- Excessive channel zapping can affect the melatonin or sleep hormone release, causing insomnia. So lack of sleep is another trigger.

This list is a conservative one. We cannot quite change all the circumstances that we are exposed to routinely. However, we can surely boost our health and ensure that we minimise the body's response to these stresses. Below are five poses that can ensure you do not fall prey to headaches.

PARVATASANA (MOUNTAIN POSE)

Method

- To be done standing.
- Take position about a foot or more from a table or chair. Place palms flat on edge of the table. Inhale.
- Exhale. Bend head towards the table, press down shoulders, and press down heels.
- Hold the pose, breathing normally.

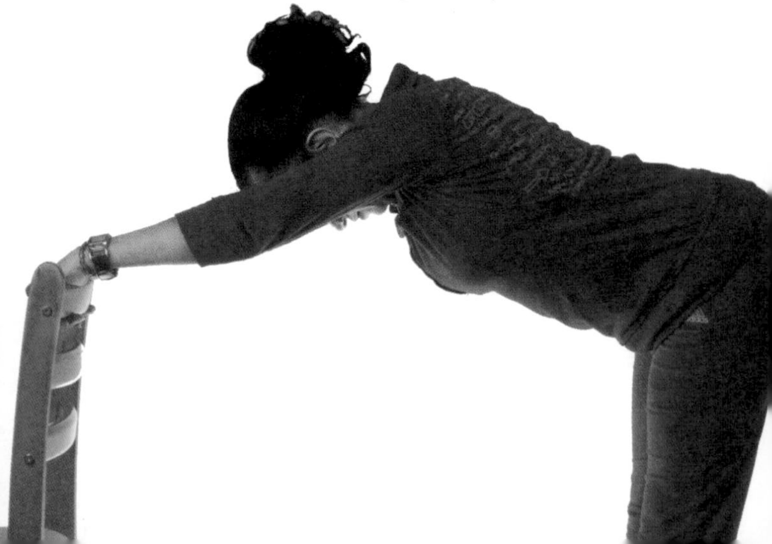

- Inhale, raise head back.
- Repeat a few times.
- After several weeks of practice do only once, but hold the final pose for longer.

How it works

- Unravels tension knots in the upper back.
- Rushes blood to the head.

Other benefits

- Relieves spinal problems, particularly of the upper back and neck region. Preventive in all back problems.
- Keeps face young and attractive due to increased blood flow to the entire face and head.
- Brain becomes alert.
- Is therapeutic in high and low blood pressure.

GOMUKH ASANA (COW-FACE POSE, WITH BOOK)

Method

- May be done seated or standing.
- Keep a heavy book ready.
- If seated on a chair, sit at the edge, leaving enough space behind for passing a book.
- Take the book in your right hand.
- Inhale. Pass the book over your right shoulder.
- Exhale, taking your left hand behind to grasp the book. Then take the book in the left hand.

- Inhale, bringing the left hand in front, passing book over left shoulder.
- Exhale, take right hand behind to grasp book and take hold of it. This completes one round.
- Do five to ten rounds.

How it works

- It releases tension from the upper back region.
- Enhances breathing, offering a subtle but powerful stress release.

Other benefits

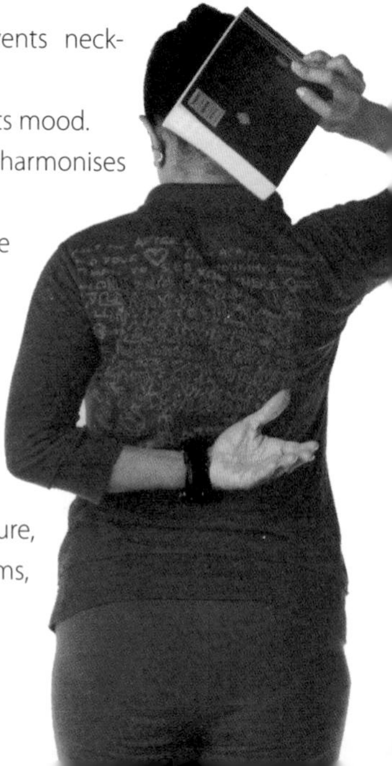

- Works upper body, prevents neck-related problems.
- Improved respiration uplifts mood.
- Improves mental focus, harmonises both brain hemispheres.
- Gives traction to the entire spine.
- Aligns the body, improving posture.
- Is a powerful cure-all pose.
- Is used as therapy in most ailments like blood pressure, diabetes, all spinal problems, respiratory ailments.

- Used in therapy for emotional issues as well, like depression or lethargy.

MARJARI ASANA (CAT STRETCH, CHAIR YOGA VERSION)

Method

- Stand or sit on the edge of a chair.
- Place hands on either hip.
- Inhale. Curve your spine, so stomach juts out. Simultaneously, lift your head towards the ceiling.
- Exhale, drop head, so chin almost touches the chest and the back rounds up.
- Tighten muscles in the stomach.
- If comfortable, hold breath for a few seconds in this position.
- Release. Repeat three to five times.

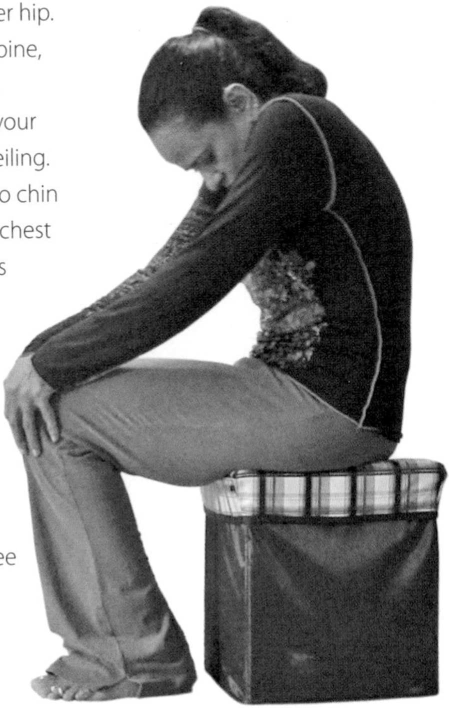

Points to note

You may hold your breath for a few seconds in the final pose, but avoid if you have epilepsy.

Other benefits

- A powerful, cure-all pose.
- Works out the entire spine.
- Boosts blood circulation to the brain.
- Heals or controls respiratory ailments.
- Calms instantly.

TRIKONASANA (TRIANGLE POSE)

Method

- Sit up straight on a chair, feet flat on the ground, knees apart.
- Inhale, hold arms out at shoulder-level.
- Exhale, twist torso to the right, bending left hand at elbow, placing it on right knee. Look up at the right hand, held aloft.
- Hold for a few seconds, breathing normally.
- Release, returning to starting position.
- Repeat thrice. Relax.
- Repeat the entire sequence for the left side.

Points to note

If you have any severe spinal problem, practise only in a phased manner.

How it works

- Releases tension locked in the upper body.
- Encourages blood flow in the 'frozen' or disused parts of the body, correcting postural defects and toning arteries.

Other benefits

- Gives a lateral stretch and traction to spine.
- Trims fat on the inner torso.
- Tones arms.
- Balances both brain hemispheres.
- Massages the liver, helping it detoxify.

MAHASIRS MUDRA (LARGE HEAD MUDRA)

Method

- Sit in a meditative fashion, eyes shut, spine erect.
- Touch the tips of the thumb with the tips of the index and middle finger.
- Press down the ring finger so it touches base of the thumb.
- Little finger should be extended.
- Do it for both hands.
- Hold for at least three to five minutes for relief. You can also do it several times during the day.

How it works

- It uses the principle of homunculus man, or the neurological map of our body in our brain, tweaking control from within.
- In ayurvedic parlance, it suppresses the lethargy-inducing earth element, while increasing the air and space element for energy.
- Relieves congestion.

Other benefits

- Increases energy levels.
- Is soothing, tension-relieving.

What else?

- Headache-relieving exercises are also tied to relieving tension. So, all poses are calming and soothing, since they **release muscular tension and emotional stress**.
- Most exercises work on the health of the **respiratory tract** since that is closely linked to headache triggers.
- These postures are mood-uplifting, and **fight depression**.
- Spinal correction and postural alignment are also tied to headache relief, hence your **carriage will improve** automatically through regular practice of these poses.
- Some of these poses are **fat-busters**, due to their effect on the liver and pancreas.

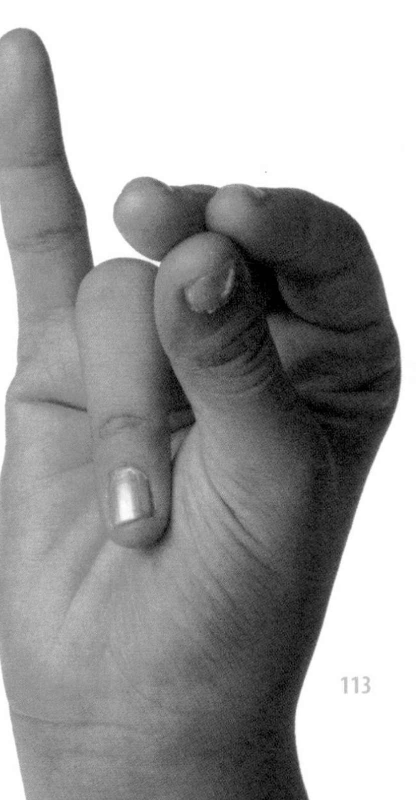

We hope that you're by now intimately aware of the anatomy of stress at work. Research proves that no one is immune to stress, neither the office-goer multi-tasking at work nor the homemaker who feels the disarray of an open-ended day and lack of challenges as acute stress. So, technically none can escape the clinging clutches of stress.

We all know it slams immunity, opening our flanks to all kinds of ailments. Stress is the trigger for most chronic ailments that lurk in our genes — high blood pressure, diabetes, cardiac mishaps, arthritis, rheumatism, migraines, ulcers and almost all digestive ailments, ranging from chronic constipation to irritable bowel syndrome, from the more embarrassing flatulence to the most discomfiting acidity and the off-putting halitosis. Respiration and our sense of control are so intimately

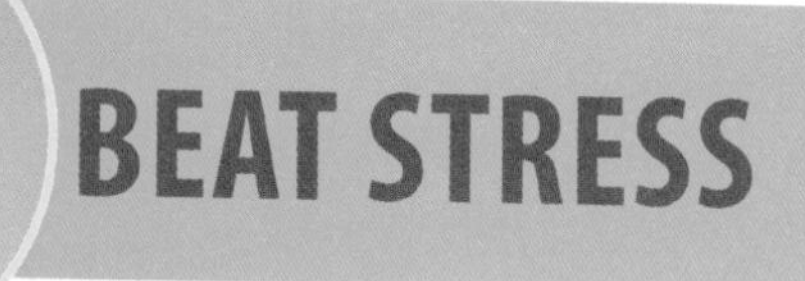

linked that you can track every breathing problem back to our stress quotient. Stress can ruin our looks, causing blotchy skin, dark circles, lay us open to all sorts of skin infections, cause unexplained psychosomatic uritcaria, dermatitis, lead us up to the hell of binge-eating and obesity, anorexia, bulimia and ungainly belly fat.

Researchers are still digging up new stress-provoked ailments that were earlier thought to have had purely physical causes. The sad part is, even those who grin and bear stress end up collapsing under its weight. The effects may take longer, but they do eventually catch up. It has been found that stoics who suppress their emotions can suffer even worse from the negative impact of stress!

Chronic fatigue, insomnia, lethargy, lack of interest, inability to innovate, anger, anxiety, clinical depression, inability to learn anything new are a few of the emotional hazards that are recognised as directly stress-related.

It is not just the nature of work or its challenges that cause stress. Long hours of commuting, lack of sleep, irregular eating habits, excessive travel, enforced sitting for long hours, bad ergonomics, jet lag, confined spaces, forced and continuous proximity to people, electromagnetic radiation and sensitivity to it from various gadgets, proximity to office gadgets, constant ringing of phones, even artificial lighting are all interpreted by the subconscious as incessant stress triggers. The last, for instance, is now known to cause mental distraction and even negatively affects productivity!

Despite knowing so much, we can do precious little to reduce the effects of stress. Apart from, of course, yoga! Yoga works simply by wringing it out of our body where it tends to get lodged. Also, it nurses the organs and systems which feel its inflictions the most. Then, the discipline of yoga helps by transforming our attitude towards stress. In fact, stress-busting poses work not just on our anatomy but also on our psychological selves.

These poses promote attitudes that can tackle stress: forward bending poses, for instance, encourage an attitude of surrender. Chest-openers work by opening us up to challenges.

UJJAYI (VICTORY BREATH)

Method

- Sit in a meditative manner.
- Inhale with a soft pressure at the throat, so you can hear a gentle snoring sound.
- Exhale, with the same sound. This comes due to closure of epiglottis.
- This completes one round.
- Do up to nine to twelve rounds.
- After sufficient practice, ensure you are inhaling and exhaling for the same length of time.

- Later, try to increase the length of your exhalation, almost doubling it.

Points to note

Avoid if you have low blood pressure or excessive depression.

How it works

- The breathing movement presses against the large wandering nerve of the parasympathetic system, acting like a switch to set off our repairing and calming mechanism.
- It works on all the body's major systems due to the above reason, rejuvenating them.
- Heals and controls all ailments for the same reason.
- Calms the mind through the rhythmic sound.

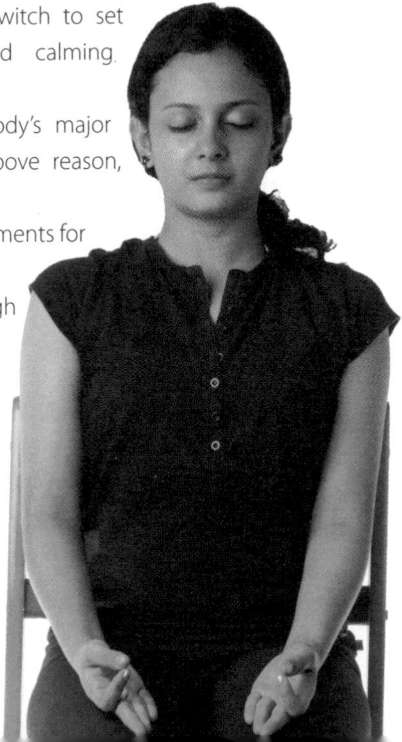

Other benefits

Is anti-ageing and beautifying.

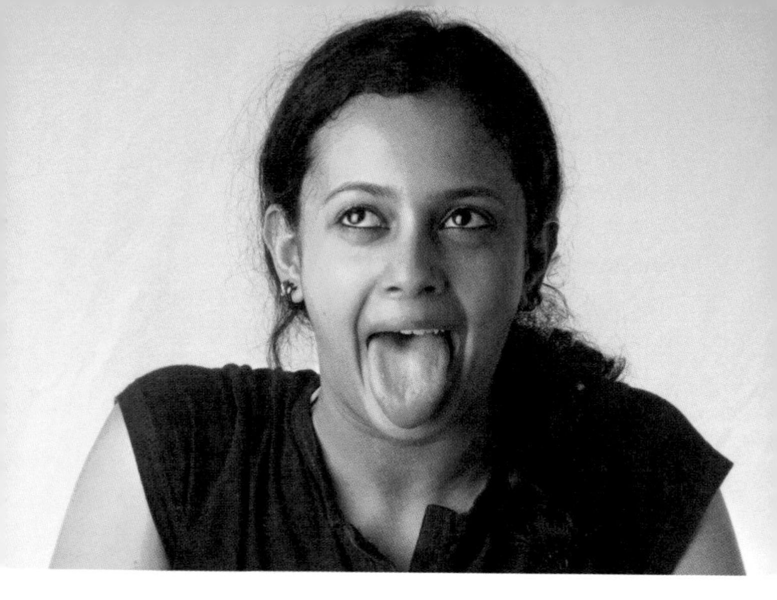

SIMHAGARJASANA (ROARING LION-FACE POSE)

Method

- To be done seated.
- Place palms flat on thighs.
- Inhale deeply.
- As you exhale, roll out tongue as far out and below as you can.
- Roll up eyes, towards ceiling.
- Ensure entire face is feeling thoroughly stretched.
- Tuck your chin lightly in.
- Hold the breath for four seconds, maintaining the pose and ensuring even the arms and legs become taut.

- Release, inhale. Then rest.
- You may repeat a few times.

Points to note

If you do not have epilepsy, heart problems or blood pressure, you can hold your breath for a count of four to ten in the final pose.

How it works

- The muscular contraction–relaxation has a powerful de-stressing effect.
- It works on the carotid sinus and other sinus hollows in the skull. This boosts the nitric oxide levels in the sensitive nasal lining. Nitric oxide not only enhances oxygen absorption but is also a well-known mood-elevator.
- Acu-points along the temple and around the eyes (Points 21 to 27) are massaged. Other acu-points along the hairline that de-stress are also worked.
- It is a powerful energiser and mood elevator.
- It has a toggle effect on blood pressure, spiking it if it is dangerously low, or lowering it when it is unhealthily high.
- It is a cure-all pose, meaning it repairs the parts of the entire body that are usually stress-hit.

Other benefits

- It works out the fifty-three facial muscles powerfully, giving them an anti-gravity workout.
- The effect on the carotid sinus ensures more oxygen intake, meaning greater facial glow.
- Acu-points (16,17,18,19, 20) running along the hair-line and temple (dealing with hair growth, vision clarity, relief in respiratory problems, removing stress, acting as face tonic) are worked out.
- Similarly, acu-points along the temples and around the eyes (21 to 27) are massaged. These deal with eye beautification, relief in nasal congestion, stress-related ailments, fighting crow's feet around the eyes and removing puffiness around the eyes. Of course, all the other points around the chin and around the nose mentioned above, are also worked out.
- It can lower fever. Relieve cold as well.

TRIKONASANA (TRIANGLE, CHAIR VERSION)

Method

- Sit on a chair, slightly towards the edge.
- Legs should be apart.
- Inhale. Spread arms out at shoulder-level.
- Exhaling, twist at the torso, towards the left.
- Simultaneously reach out right hand to touch left foot.
- Left hand is raised up. Gaze at left hand.

- Hold for a few seconds, breathing normally.
- Release. Return to starting position.
- Repeat a few times.
- Relax and repeat entire sequence for the other side.

How it works

- It massages the adrenal glands, involved intimately with stress.
- The shoulders, the upper body, neck are regions where stress is felt as muscular contractions. The exercise wrings out such biological impacts of stress.
- The head, which normally experiences reduced blood flow when there is excessive stress, gets a gentle gush of blood.
- Respiration, which is deeply and negatively impacted by stress, is boosted.

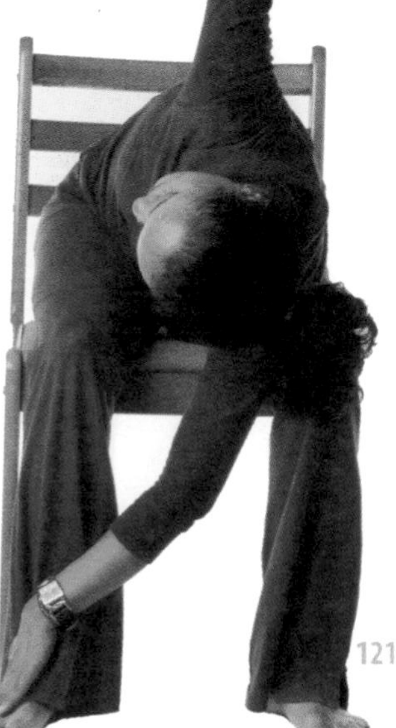

Other benefits

- Squeezes the liver, aiding the release of fat.
- Tones spine and nerves.
- Improves posture.
- Promotes mental focus.

NATVARASANA (LORD KRISHNA POSE)

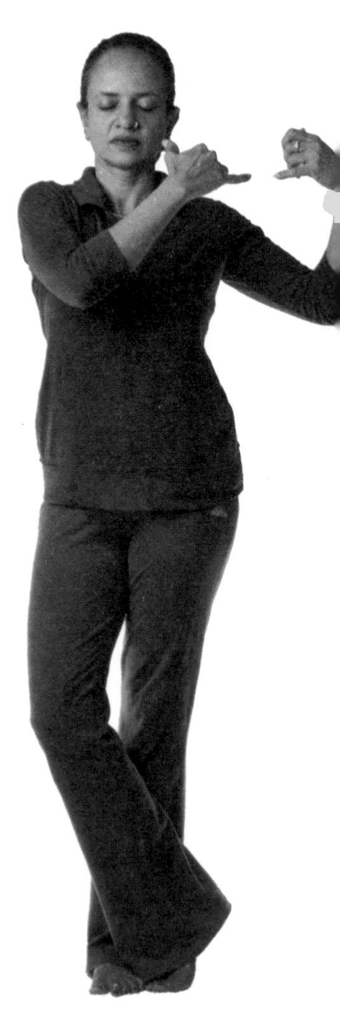

Method

Stand up straight. Pass right foot over left foot. Place toes of your right foot beside the left foot. Ensure feet are close to each other. Hold hands towards the left (as shown in the picture alongside), as if holding a flute. Shut your eyes. Hold the pose to a count of thirty. Release. Repeat the entire sequence for the other side.

Benefits

Balances both sides of the body. Also harmonises both brain hemispheres helping us achieve mental balance. Improves confidence, removes shyness and social anxiety. Tones nerves.

HASTA UTTANASANA (HAND-RAISING POSE)

Method

- Sit on a chair. Inhale. Exhale.
- Inhaling, pass both arms over the back rest.
- Remain seated in this pose for a few seconds, feeling the chest expand.
- Interlock fingers, inhale.
- Exhale. Inhaling, lift arms gently as much as you can, to extend the stretch.
- Release with an exhalation, dropping arms back gently.
- Repeat a few times.

Points to note

- Avoid in case of cardiac problems, though the exercise may be learned in a phased manner, under guidance.
- This exercise may be done standing as well with hands interlocked behind. If your office chair has a wide back rest, you may not be comfortable doing it seated. It would be better to do the standing version then.

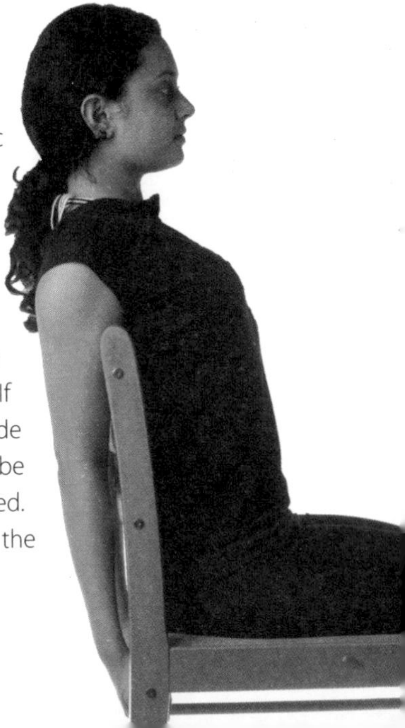

How it works

- The chest expansion has a liberating effect through enhanced breathing.
- This pose boosts mood and energy levels.
- The 'stress spots' of neck, upper back, shoulder are massaged gently, so the unconscious contractions in the areas are undone.

Other benefits

- Arms are toned.
- Improves posture.

What else?

- These are **detox poses**, which power your day by removing accumulated waste and toxins.
- They rejuvenate by flushing the entire body-mind complex with a fresh shot of energy. They are **mood-elevators**.
- All poses, especially simhagarjasana (lion-roaring), ujjayi pranayama (victory breath), natvarasana (Krishna pose), are **anti-ageing and beautifying**. They will not only de-stress but give you that **yogic glow.**

You know smoking is injurious to health. Well, physical inactivity can be more injurious than smoking. It has been found that thirty-five per cent of cardiovascular problems arise due to inactivity. A passive lifestyle also contributes to diabetes, high blood pressure, high cholesterol, obesity, addictive behaviour — all of which cause or accompany cardiovascular problems.

Inactivity induces less compliance from arteries (simply meaning you are in for a cardiac problem) and more insulin resistance (linked to diabetes mellitus). In fact, this connection was found even in younger people, overturning the earlier belief that ageing and cardiovascular problems were related. Research has found that inactivity can make us biologically older.

Since belly fat and obesity are closely linked to cardiovascular disasters, activity that factors in weight loss

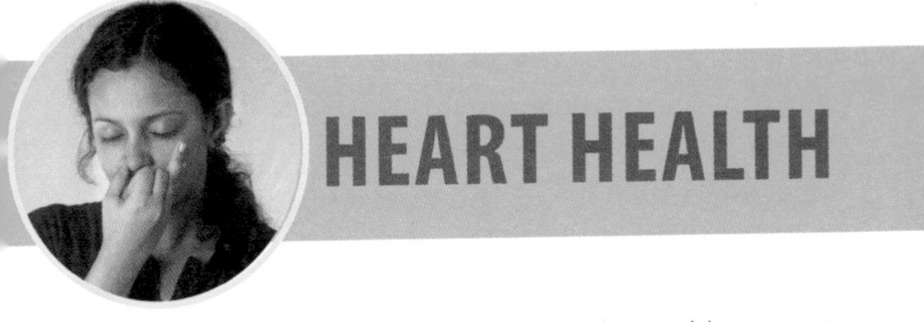

is absolutely important. Cardiovascular problems start when deposits begin to line the arteries, putting extra pressure on the heart to pump the blood to the rest of the body. The heart pumps about 7,000 litres of blood daily;

it could do well with a little consideration and help from your side!

Though many of you would like a passive lifestyle because you believe it gives your heart rest, the heartbeat depends a lot on your emotional response to stress. So, having an exercise regime that sensitises you to your heartbeat and builds up its endurance levels to new highs is very crucial if you want it to beat for a long time.

Healthy blood vessels are elastic. When they lose tone, you are in for a major, unpleasant cardiovascular surprise. This is because the inner linings of the blood vessels, called endothelium, has cells that are extremely cued-in to signals from your thoughts, what you eat, your activity levels, your muscular needs. When they are efficient, they accommodate all those demands your body and mind places on them: but when they are inefficient due to any of the above causes (bad diet, obesity, inactivity) they can cut down blood flow drastically, making the heart struggle that much more.

But beyond the life-and-death issue of the heart, the circulatory system is tied up with other systems too. It decides your skin's tone and youthfulness. It can decide the lustre of your hair. It is blood that transports oxygen in the body; the sense of lethargy and fatigue can be directly linked to our circulatory system's own dullness. Even eating healthy is not relevant if your digestive system (which again depends on the blood) is not able to efficiently absorb the nutrients that entered through your mouth. Your mood swings, the transport of hormones, the communication of your brain cells — all ultimately depend on your circulatory system. Keeping it happy is not just about health. It is about the harmony we all crave and work for.

Below are a few yogic moves to help it get back on track. These simple yogic moves will instantly relax and calm you. Use them to hyperventilate irritation or stress at work, and keep your blood-flow smooth.

PRANAM MUDRA (PRAYER GESTURE)

Method

- May be done standing or seated.
- Keep the spine erect.

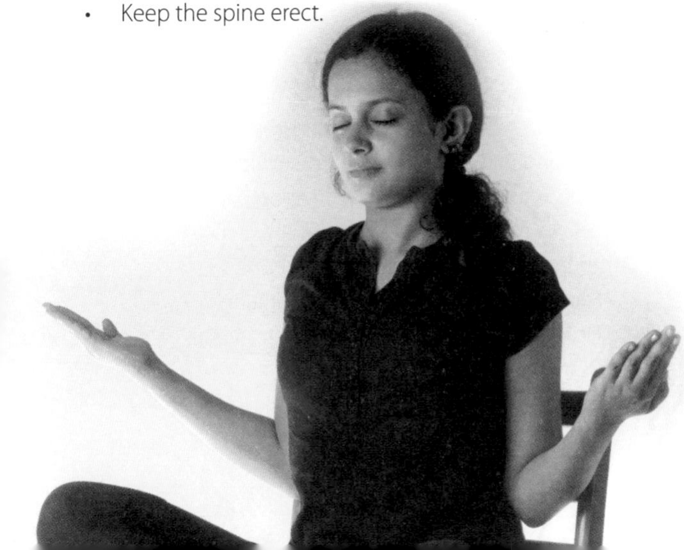

- Inhale. Spread arms at shoulder level, palms facing upward.
- Exhaling, lower them gently, so the elbows rest on the waist.
- Lower arms jut out, on either side of the waist.
- Hold for a few seconds, breathing normally.
- Relax hands, before raising them back to starting position, repeat five to ten times.

Points to note

- The slower the breath and each motion, the deeper the relaxation.
- In the final pose, keeping the torso erect and the palms aligned with your body will enhance the positive impact on breath and mood.

How it works

- All hand movements that work the chest and expand it are known to boost the heart's health.
- This pose is a powerful de-stresser, helping to calm you and relieve anxiety or stress which often disrupts the circulatory system by increasing palpitations, etc.

Other benefits

- Expands the chest, boosting respiration.
- Fights depression.
- Removes lethargy.
- Works upper body, easing frozen shoulders.

NADI SHUDDI (CLEANSING BREATH)

Method

- Pranayamas, or breathing exercises, are best done seated.
- Shut eyes. Keeping eyes shut during pranayama keeps the mind focused.
- Fold down right index finger and middle finger.
- The thumb and the other two fingers that remain extended are used to close and open your nostrils on right and left respectively. Press your right nostril down with your thumb and inhale from left.
- Using the extended fingers, shut both nostrils for a few seconds.

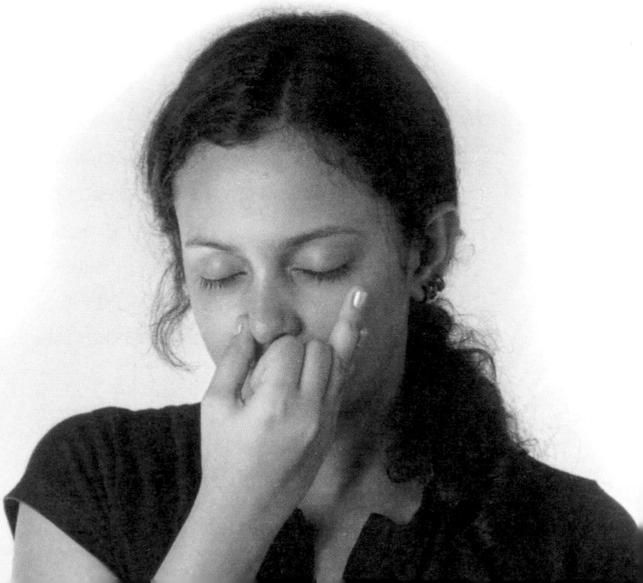

- Lift your right thumb off the right nostril and exhale.
- Now inhale from the right.
- Hold both nostrils for some time, using fingers as suggested above.
- Exhale from the left.
- This is one round. Do up to five to nine rounds.

Points to note

- Slowly, after some practice, you may introduce counts: inhaling to a count of four and exhaling to a count of six and retaining breath to a count of four.
- The counts given are very minimal. As you advance, attend some pranayama course to extend your capacity in this aspect.
- This is one of the few exercises without too many contraindications; it is a cure-all one.

How it works

- The hand position suggested is called Vishnu mudra and is said to impact the cardiac plexus powerfully, through acupressure points. This exercise purifies energy channels, seen as the main cause for most diseases of the mind and body. Despite its simplicity, this is the most important and most therapeutic of all yogic practices.

Other benefits

- It is used as therapy for all major ailments of the body, such as heart diseases, cancer, arthritis, etc.
- It is also the best therapy in most mind-related problems: psychosomatic disorders, depression, panic attacks, anger.

SUKRI MUDRA (CURE-ALL HAND GESTURE)

Method

- Sit up straight.
- Shut eyes.
- Touch the tip of all four fingers to tip of the thumb.
- Do this for both hands. Place hands on thighs.
- Hold for three to five minutes.

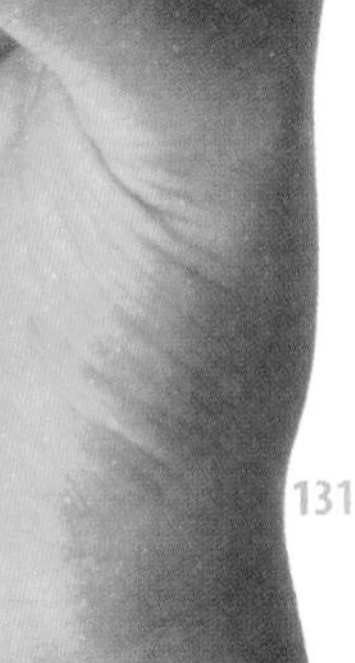

How it works

- As explained elsewhere, this (like other mudras/ hand gestures) works on the neurological map of our body parts in the brain, tweaking them to function for our benefit.

Other benefits

- It balances all the three doshas.
- Removes sluggishness.
- Is therapeutic in anxiety and anger.
- Works on all the major systems, restoring and healing them.
- Is also a preventive in most physical and emotional ailments.

HASTA UTTANASANA (HAND-RAISING POSE)

Method

- Sit on a chair. May also be done standing.
- Keep your back straight. Inhale.
- Hold arms out, at shoulder level, so they are parallel to the ground.
- Exhale. Inhaling, push back palms, as if swimming the breast stroke.
- Move palms back and forth five to ten times.

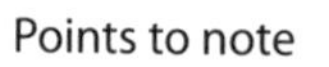

Points to note

Ensure body remains straight throughout.

Other benefits

- Opens up the chest, expanding the rib cage, facilitating and boosting natural breath capacity.
- This in turn boosts one's mood immediately.

- The immune gland at the chest is also massaged, boosting your ability to fight infections and serious problems, like cancer.
- Posture is superbly aligned, rectifying and preventing spinal problems.

KASHTATAKSHANSANA (WOOD-CHOPPING POSE)

Method

- Sit on a chair (may also be done standing).
- Inhale, interlock both hands.
- Exhale to stretch interlocked hands in front.
- Inhale, lifting interlocked hands high, overhead. Exhale, bring both hands down swiftly and vigorously, with a chopping motion.
- This is one round. Do ten to fifteen rounds, with breath awareness.

How it works

- Hand movements and the heart's well-being are linked. This pose works out the heart and the circulatory system powerfully.

Other benefits

- Breath awareness with this repetitive motion improves mental focus.
- Upper body is toned, with shoulder joints getting a powerful workout.
- Prevents frozen shoulder and neck pains.
- Since shoulder muscles also support the respiratory system, breathing is enhanced powerfully, in turn lifting the mood.

What else?

- These yogic practices work out the pectorals (chest muscles), **improving overall posture and carriage**. Toned muscles in the torso will make you look svelte, also taking the weight off your overburdened legs by propping the spine.

- The hand movements help in **lengthening and deepening the breath**, boosting lung volume.
- All chest exercises also **boost immunity**.
- Chest exercises spike one's mood by encouraging **psycho-physical extroversion.**

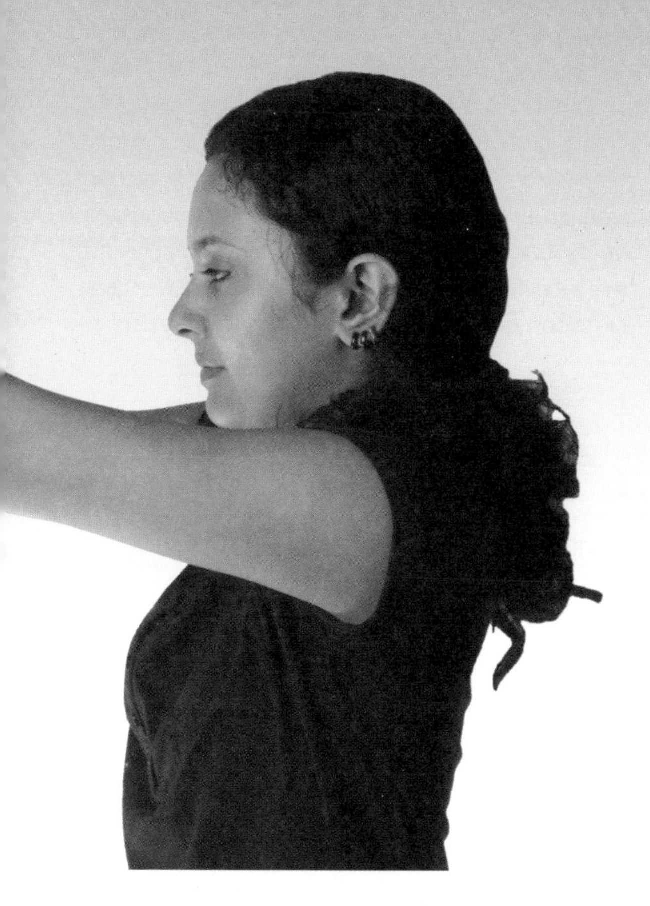

Some lifestyle-related facts are well known and some well established. By now everybody knows that smokers are at a high risk of lung cancer. What is not so well-known, but well established, is the link between a passive lifestyle and Type 2 diabetes. We are genetically prone to it! Indians suffer the unfortunate ranking as the ethnic group most prone to diabetes. Plus our sedentary lifestyle makes us even more susceptible to the disease.

Since diabetes is also linked to heart ailments, other circulatory problems such as stroke, uro-genital complications (kidney disease, impotence or erectile dysfunction), eye problems (like glaucoma and loss of eye-sight), fungal infections of foot and skin (operations become difficult on those with a high blood sugar count due to post-operation complications) and a nerve debility

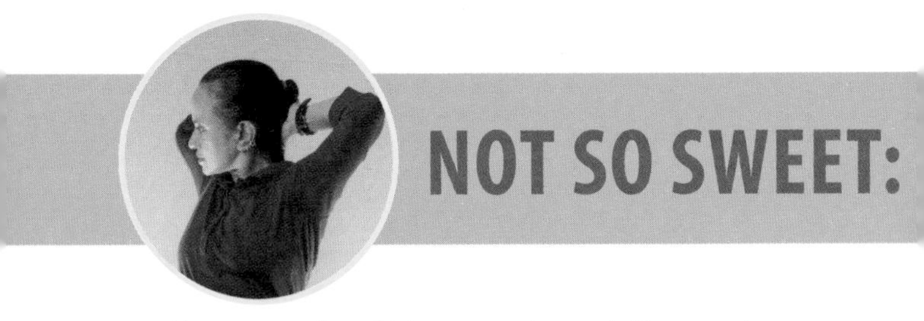

NOT SO SWEET:

like neuropathy which can restrict one's life severely.

It goes without saying that once the body gets accustomed to a passive lifestyle, it finds any form of activity irksome and resists it; those with a sedentary work-style invariably choose recreation which is passive, like watching television. It is not far-fetched to assume that this habit also has its own eating patterns and habits which are considered unhealthy — comfort eating, eating without being aware of how much or what one is eating, snacking continuously or sipping addictive drinks, whether it is alcohol or aerated drinks.

Research has shown how prolonged hours in front of the television (even amongst those who exercise) can lead to Type 2 diabetes. Some link has also been established between the lack of Vitamin D (from being confined within closed spaces for most of the day) and diabetes. Whether the inability to handle an overload of stress is the cause or symptom of diabetes is a matter of debate. However, along with this stress overdose is the ungainly addition of belly-fat, since abdominal fat is most common amongst the stress-prone. Other links that are

closely associated to diabetes are emotional ailments like depression, anxiety and irritability.

Interestingly, out of all the ailments, diabetes responds fastest to yoga therapy. However, regularity of practice is also of paramount importance. In a person with diabetes, the effect of exercise (or yoga) lasts up to a maximum of a day or two. After that, unless you maintain your regimen, you are most likely to see a relapse in the control you learnt to exert through yoga. These exercises are therefore designed to ensure that you continue to check diabetes or prevent even the pre-diabetes or metabolic syndrome (which comes with its own bouquet of ailments) even while at your desk.

PARIVRITTI KONASANA (TWISTED ANGLE POSE)

Method

- To be done seated in a chair.
- Place right hand along the chair's leg.
- Inhale. Hold left hand aloft,
- so that inner left arm touches the left ear.
- Exhale, slide right hand along the chair's leg, so that the hand reaches, or almost reaches, the ground. Left hand remains touching the ear, and becomes parallel to the ground. (See image) Breathe normally.
- Inhale, look from under the left hand

towards the ceiling, twisting torso lightly. This intensifies the stretch.

- Hold the pose, breathing normally. Release by sliding right hand back and up and raising torso to starting position.
- Do a few times.
- Rest before repeating for the other side.

Points to note

This is a powerful stretch, so ideally follow it after some light waist twists or shoulder flexes.

How it works

- It massages and rejuvenates the pancreas.
- It works out the entire digestive tract.
- Offers emotional relief by untangling the tension knots from the body.
- It is also de-stressing due to the massaging effect on adrenals or stress glands.

Other benefits

- Gives a transverse twist to the spine, toning spinal nerves and preventing spinal problems.
- Trims belly fat.
- Is mood uplifting.
- Tones liver, encouraging stored fat release.

KATI CHAKRASANA (ABDOMINAL TWIST)

Method

- May be done standing or seated.
- Fold each arm at elbow.
- Interlock hands behind back of head, the arms still folded.
- Inhale. Exhaling twist body to the right. Adjust elbows so they remain straight out.
- Inhale, return to the centre.
- Exhale, twist to the left.
- This completes one round.
- Do three to five rounds.

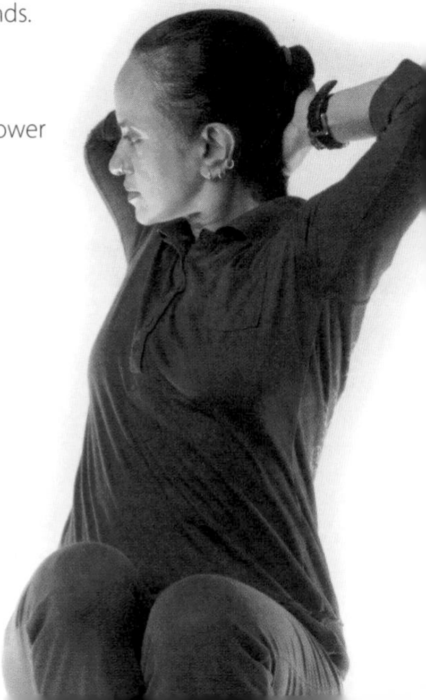

Points to note

Avoid if having lower backache.

How it works

As explained above.

Other benefits

- Preventive in spinal problems.
- Trims fat along the torso, especially stomach.

- Boosts digestion, encourages fat-release from liver.
- Relieves constipation.
- Is uplifting.

UTTHITA MARICHYASANA (RAISED SAGE MARICHAYA POSE)

Method

- Stand up straight, with a chair on your right.
- Bend right leg to place right foot on the chair seat. Foot must be pointing to the right.
- Place arms at shoulder level. Bend at elbows. Ensure elbows are not sagging.
- Inhale. Exhaling, twist torso and face the right side.
- Hold for a few seconds, breathing normally.
- Inhale to return to starting position.
- Do a few times.
- Rest. Then repeat for the other side.

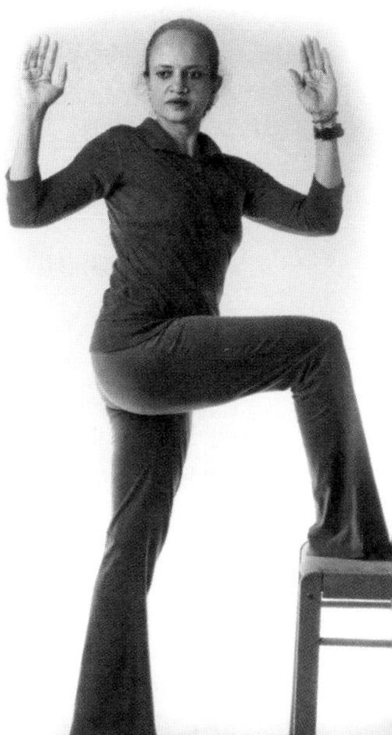

Points to note

- The extent of your twist will depend on your flexibility. So do not strain, but consistently and deliberately extend this with regular, daily practice.

- For enhanced benefits, learn to hold the final twist for longer after a few weeks of regular practice.

How it works

Poses that apply abdominal pressure have powerful therapeutic value in diabetes management because they massage the pancreas (involved with blood sugar management), the stress glands or adrenals (which are delicately linked to blood sugar levels) and the digestive tract.

Other benefits

- Preventive in spinal problems and helps relieve existing ones.
- Fights fat.
- Tones legs.
- Is detoxifying, due to impact on liver.
- Boosts digestion, metabolism.
- Is therapeutic in most ailments.

ARDHA TITALI (HALF BUTTERFLY POSE)

Method

- Sit on a chair with both feet flat on the ground in front.
- Bend right leg, place back of right foot on left thigh.
- Place the foot as high as possible.
- Inhale. Exhaling, hug the right knee to chest.

- Inhale, drop the knee back. Press it down with right hand.
- This is one round.
- Do up to ten rounds.
- Then repeat for the other leg.

How it works

- The pressure at the abdomen has all the benefits and impacts mentioned above.

Other benefits

- It is a preparatory pose, getting you flexible and fit for advanced poses.
- It is therapeutic in most ailments.
- It opens up the hips, also affecting the glands in this region. Particular impact is on the uro-genital set, affecting the state of well-being also.

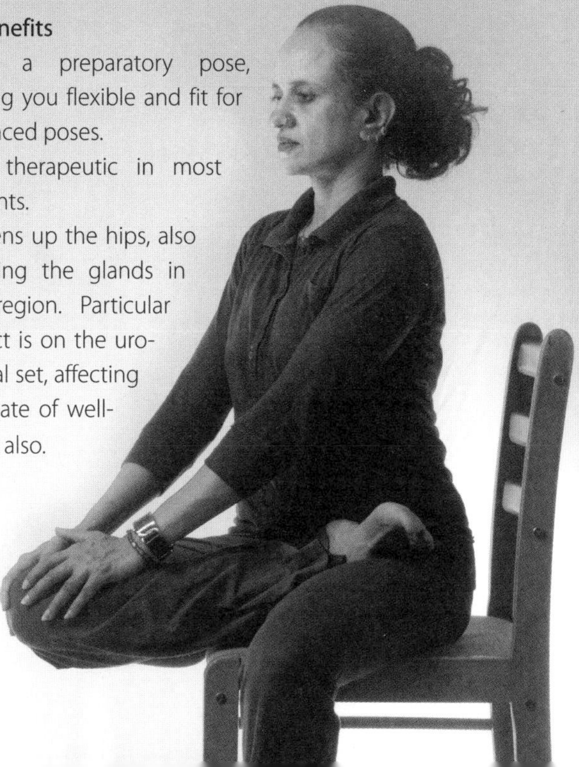

KAPALABHATI PRANAYAMA (SKULL-CLEANSING BREATHING PRACTICE)

Method

- Sit up straight.
- Shut eyes.
- Keep hands in any common mudra (or surya mudra, explained earlier in the chapter on obesity).
- Inhale and exhale consciously for a few seconds.
- After a deep inhalation, begin to exhale forcefully and continuously.
- Do this fast, counting up to thirty exhalations.
- Stop. Breathe normally. This is one round.
- Repeat twice.

Points to note

- Avoid if having high blood pressure, heart ailments, ulcers, other inflammatory conditions like fever, irritable bowel syndrome.

- It is a stimulating practice, so avoid practising it close to bed-time, since it will affect sleep by keeping your mind alert.
- After a few months of regular practice, you can increase the number of beats/exhalations for each round slowly, up to sixty.

How it works

As explained above.

Other benefits

- Aids weight loss.
- Stimulates mind. Is used to treat depression.
- Removes sluggishness, daytime sleepiness.
- Tightens abdomen.
- Relieves headaches.
- Is therapeutic in respiratory problems.

What else?

- All these exercises, since they work on the abdomen so powerfully and tweak metabolism, are also **weight-loss aids**.
- They also prevent and **rectify postural defects and abdominal sagging**.
- Since they work on the adrenal or stress glands, their impact on **stress control** is immediate and effective.
- All are **mood-elevators.**

Most people think they fall ill largely due to external reasons. For them the very idea that they may be partly contributing to their own weakened immune system may come as an unpleasant and unacceptable surprise. It nevertheless happens to be true.

Here are some hard-hitting facts that should explain how we are our own worst enemy!

- Exercise or motion propels immune cells around the body more quickly to protect us. When we are sedentary, we deny ourselves this armour plating.
- While casual exercise or movement assures this, it has to be consistent. Sporadic exercise offers only 'part-time' effects.
- The wrong type of exercise can make one even more susceptible to infections, because the body is stressed and the immune system dips dangerously due to

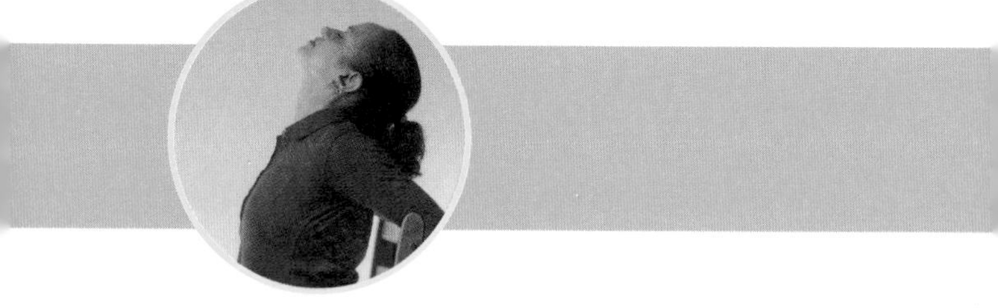

hormonal shifts caused by misguided exercises.
- On the other hand, a well-crafted exercise programme (like yoga or moderate gym exercise) enhances lymphatic activity. Lymphatic fluid helps transport

white blood cells (or our defence squad) to body sites that need them to fight infections. They also remove dead bacteria and damaged cells. Since the lymphatic system depends entirely on muscular activity to pump this lymphatic fluid around, exercise or physical activity that works your entire body is crucial for your health.

- The thymus gland, which is as big as the heart in children, begins to shrink as people grow older, further affecting the production of immune T cells needed to fight infections. However, this shrinkage is reversible and responds positively to exercise.

As you can see, if you do not exercise, you are bound to fall ill. The connection is simple. Being work-bound can no longer be cited as an excuse for shirking exercise: to remain at your desk longer, you must learn to move your body right, throughout the day. You simply cannot be

an effective or efficient worker otherwise, if you become susceptible to every passing infection.

Below are powerful yogic poses which massage the thymus gland and work the body to set off lymphatic activity that will keep you buzzing with health at work.

ARDHA USHTRASANA (HALF CAMEL)

Method

- Sit on a chair sideways.
- Press feet down or point toes to floor, if your feet do not reach.
- Press down hips on chair. Inhale, raising right hand up, in front of you, at shoulder level.
- Exhale.
- Inhaling, gently drop head back, curving the spine inwards.
- Hold for a few seconds, breathing normally, focusing your attention on the right hand.
- Release. Repeat a few times.
- Relax, before repeating the sequence for the left hand.

Points to note

Avoid dropping your neck back if you have severe neck pain or vertigo. You may gently expand your chest without dropping the head back for similar, though reduced, impact.

How it works

- It expands the chest, powerfully working the thymus gland.
- The shoulder region also gets a workout. This is essential since lymph nodes from here and the neck are involved in releasing fluids that transport the

immune cells around.

- The enhanced breathing also boosts overall health.

Other benefits

- By opening up the chest, this pose revs up lung capacity.
- It boosts circulation in the entire torso, even impacting metabolism and weight loss in general.
- Is preventive in shoulder problems.
- Boosts mood.

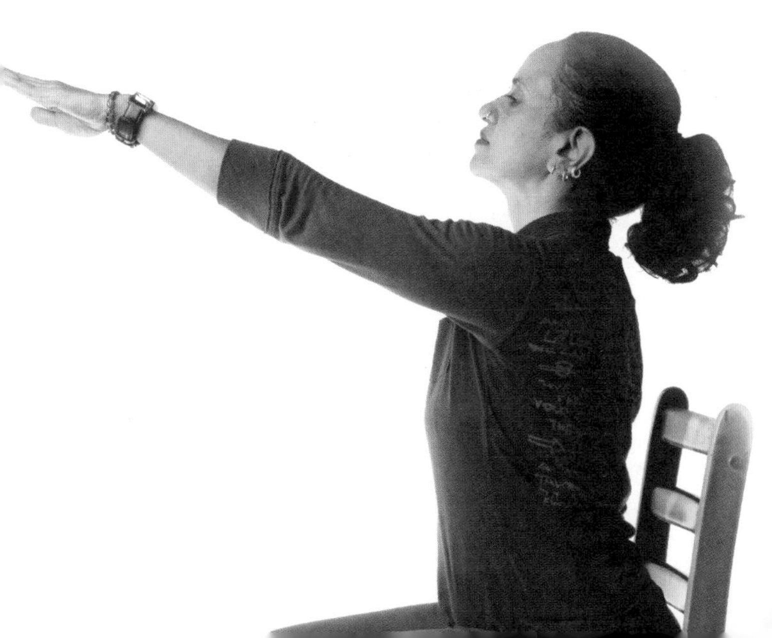

USHTRASANA (CAMEL POSE)

Method

- Sit on chair, as in previous exercise.
- Place both hands back, to grasp chair rim from behind.
- Inhale, tilting head gently backwards and arching spine inwards.
- Hold the pose, breathing normally.
- Release to return to starting position. Repeat a few times.

Points to note

As above.

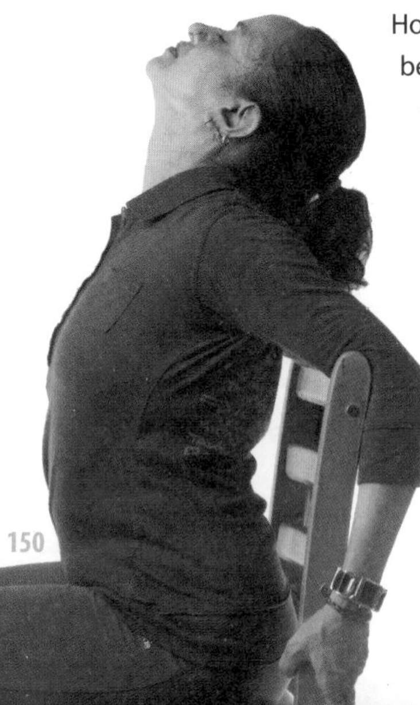

How it works and other benefits

- Same as above, more enhanced.
- As a stimulating practice, it also aids weight loss, pepping respiratory rate, hiking metabolism.
- Is preventive in neck pain.

SKANDA CHAKRA (SHOULDER ROLL)

Method

- Done seated or standing.
- Inhale, move shoulders up, towards ears.
- Drop them back with an exhalation.
- Do five to ten times.

How it works

- It works the shoulder region which, as we explained above, is also involved closely with immune activity.
- The chest also gets a subtle up-down workout that further manipulates the thymus.

Other benefits

- Is preventive and healing in neck pain.
- Encourages blood flow in the upper torso.
- Opens up chest, enhancing respiration by working the muscles that support respiration in the neck and shoulders.

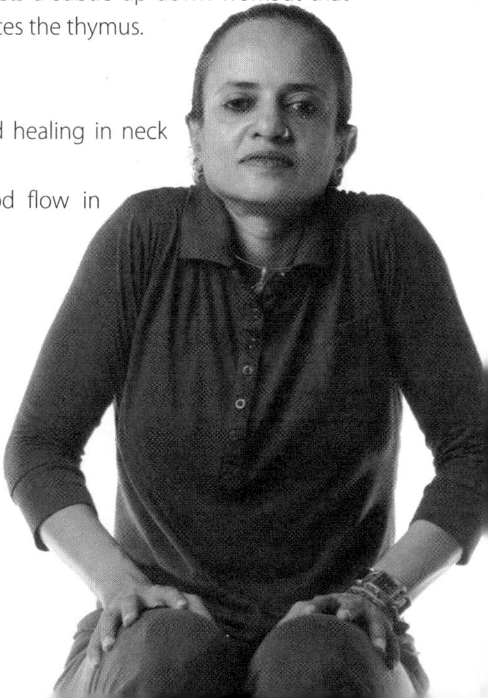

- Relieves frozen shoulders.
- Is a powerful de-stressing practice, since it unknots stress tangles from this region, which get contracted with tension.

MERU PRISHTASANA (SPINE POSE)

Method

- Done seated or standing.
- Inhale. Exhaling, bring shoulders in front, so chest caves in.
- Inhale, expand chest, driving the rib cage out and up, by pushing back shoulders.
- This is one round. Do up to ten rounds.

How it works and other benefits

- Same as above, but more enhanced.
- It is a mood-uplifting pose.
- Improves confidence.
- Removes lethargy.

TRIKAYA TADASANA

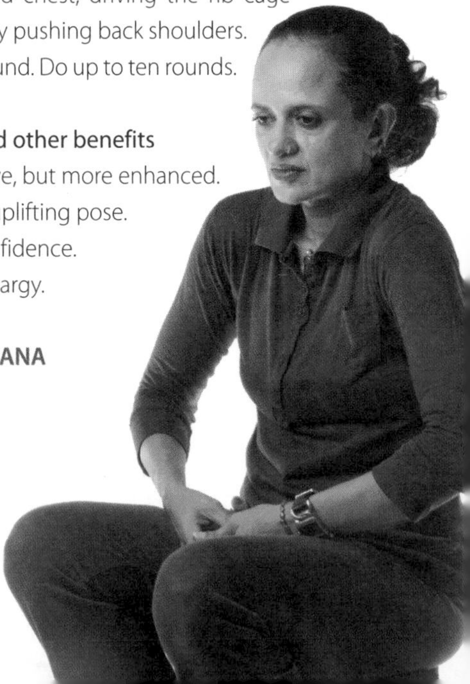

(SWAYING PALM TREE POSE)

Method

- May be done seated or standing.
- Raise both hands, interlocking fingers. Inhale.
- Exhaling, bend head and arms towards the left. Torso also bends towards the left. Feel the stretch along entire right side.
- Hold this pose, breathing normally.
- Return to centre, inhaling.
- This is one round.
- Do ten to fifteen rounds.

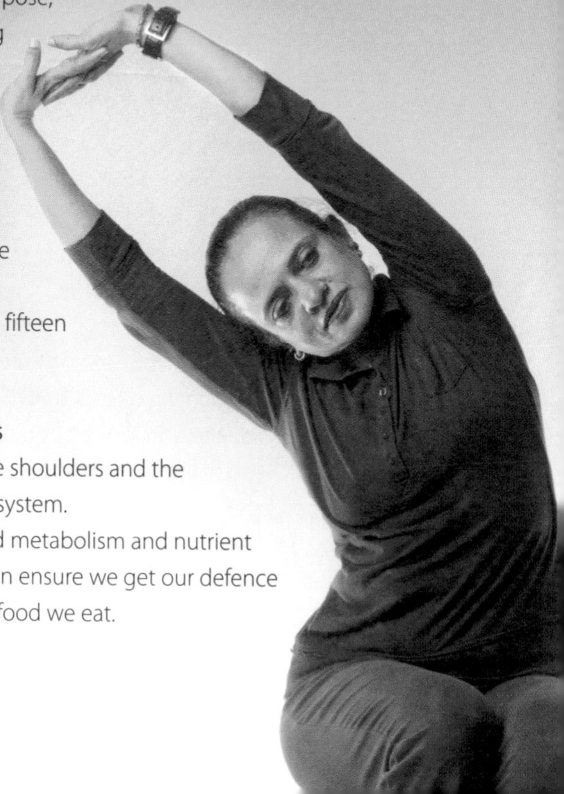

How it works

- Works the shoulders and the immune system.
- Enhanced metabolism and nutrient absorption ensure we get our defence from the food we eat.

- Enhanced breathing further armour-plates us by improving overall ability to deal with stress.
- By de-stressing powerfully it removes the damage and vulnerability that tension causes within our body's healing systems.

Other benefits

- Trims arms.
- Trims legs as well if done standing.
- Gives traction to the spine, preventing spinal problems. Is therapeutic in most spinal ailments, especially upper body.
- Uplifts emotionally.
- Boosts respiration.
- Is used to control blood pressure problems and diabetes, the latter due to pressure on the pancreas.

What else?

- Backbends and side-bends in yoga are a great way to revive a flagging day. They **boost one's mood**. This happens due to enhanced respiration and blood circulation — so many good things in one stroke. Do these yogic back bends to perk up your work day.
- Strong chest muscles not only add to the aesthetic appeal of our body, but support **efficient respiration**. This is preventive in most respiratory problems.

- The subtle pressure also works out and improves **heart stamina**.
- Chest openers are **emotionally extroverting**. They remove shyness.
- They improve our voice, thus powering our **communication skills** by working on the throat region and the neck region involved with voice transfer and throw.
- They also **de-stress superbly**, by releasing the tension knots from the upper body.
- They also work the facial muscles, keeping us **looking young** by pushing back lines around the eyes and mouth due to the tautness they cause.

Several research studies, including those conducted in India, have shown that, increasingly, young people are having problems related to the uro-genital system. Infertility, low libido, impotence, erectile dysfunction, hormonal upsets (more common with women) and kidney woes are afflicting even the youth now.

While everybody points a finger at the omnipresent villain called stress, other factors are also being examined as triggers. An increasingly sedentary way of working and living, lack of exercise, over-exposure to electromagnetic radiation (from gadgets), excessive use of computers, which encourages postural defects that also ruin pelvic tone, and wrong eating habits are amongst a few.

Here are some other suspects that you may have unwittingly invited into your lifestyle:

- Anti-depressants like Prozac (interestingly, some drugs increase sexual appetite but mar ability to perform!)

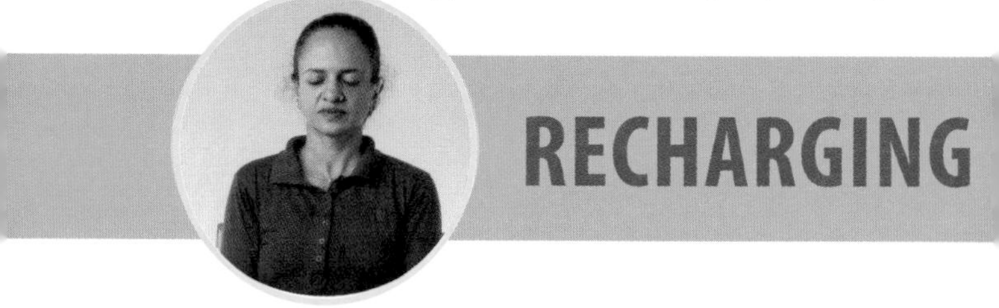

  and sedatives are big culprits. Others include 'quack' diet pills, anti-seizure drugs and anti-hypertensives used to lower blood pressure, including some beta-blockers and diuretics.

- Preservatives in packaged food (innocently labelled nitrates, such as sodium nitrates) do a reverse-Viagra act! Meaning they block blood vessels to sexual organs, causing erectile dysfuntion in men and impairing clitoral stimulation in women. Also, the subversive food additive monosodium glutamate (used in fast food and Chinese takeaways), is a sex depressant.
- Alcohol, contrary to common perception, does not lead to greater appetite for sex. In moderation, it excites. Excessively, it affects the brain's GABA receptors (these inhibit the brain cell action) and disrupts the sensitive orchestration between the sympathetic and para-sympathetic nervous systems crucial for procreation, apart from directly affecting changes in sex hormonal flow. It also siphons off zinc, magnesium and vitamin Bs needed for a robust sex

life.
- That dirty word 'stress' again. Neurotransmitters or brain messengers like norepinephrine, serotonin, dopamine and histamine are crucial for focusing on any task. Since these are also involved with sexual

activity, any mental distraction, including stress and overwork, is likely to jar their delicate symphony of sexual pleasure.

In case you're thinking you'll be able to catch up on your sexual life later on, you may still want to watch against mess-ups with this system. Why? Because problems here also mean problems elsewhere.

Such as: • You may stop enjoying food for a while, as taste buds deaden. • You could suffer from chronic headaches. • Chronic fatigue will also plague you. • Urinary infections tend to become commonplace, including painful urination. • Water retention may become commonplace, meaning that awful bloating sensation that also makes you look bloated. • High blood pressure. • Skin problems, including pigmentation or itchiness. • Depression. • Low enthusiasm. • Insomnia. • Memory failure. • Osteoporosis.

Here are a few yogic tricks to get this fussy system back on track. Also, take a look at your diet and see if any of these is missing from your daily menu: 'Happy' nutrients including vitamin Bs, manganese, magnesium, folic acids found in soya and all lentils, cabbage, wheat germ, yoghurt, bananas, whole wheat, oats, almonds and other nuts like walnuts, brown rice, sweet potatoes and sesame seeds.

KALIASANA (GODDESS KALI POSE)

Method

- Stand up straight with your feet about two-feet apart.
- Inhale, placing palms one on top of the other. Hands are held at stomach-level, in front of the navel.
- Exhaling, lower yourself so that you are fully squatting.
- Hands may touch the floor.
- Hold the pose, breathing normally.
- Inhaling, raise yourself back to the starting position. Repeat three to five times.

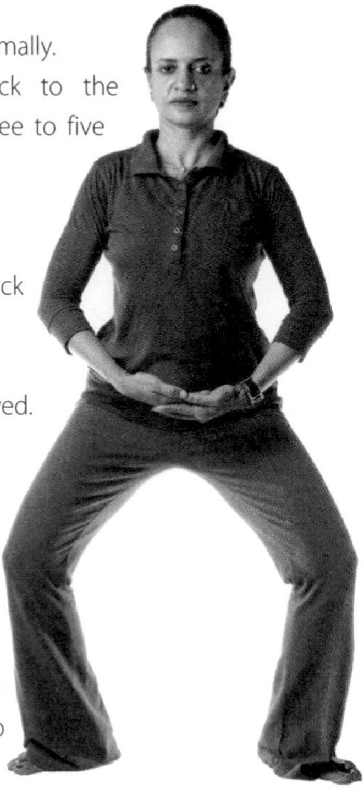

Points to note

- Avoid if you have a lower back problem.
- Beginners may only squat partially till flexibility is achieved.

How it works

- It tones the pelvis, including the floor muscles.
- Works out the entire uro-genital system.
- Tones the spine, releasing stiffness, which also compresses the uro-genital

system through bad posture.

Other benefits

- Is an energy-releasing pose.
- Tones your nerves, de-stressing you.
- Works out the entire spine.
- Trims and shapes the stomach.
- Aids weight loss.

MANDUKASANA (FROG POSE)

Method

- To be done seated.
- Sit well back in chair, bring knees together.
- Feet may point outwards, with the balls of the feet on the ground and heels slightly lifted off the ground.
- Place palms one on top of the other on your lap. Or assume the pran mudra (Page 164) to combine two practices.
- Push the hips down firmly against chair seat.
- Perineum (or groin region) should rest firmly on seat of chair.
- Focus eyes on nose tip.

Points to note

Don't strain while focusing your eyes, since this is contraindicated in severe eye problems, including cataract and glaucoma. This focus, called manduki mudra, is a precursor to meditation.

How it works

- The perineum pressure impacts the mooladhara chakra (yogic centre of creative and animal instincts).
- The focus on the nose penetrates the brain's centre for smell, the most primitive of human senses, impacting a person's subconscious drives and passions.
- Deeply calming, this shores creative energies otherwise dissipated by distractions. Hence also therapeutic in impotency and infertility.

UTTHITA PARSVAKONASANA (EXTENDED SIDE STRETCH)

Method

- Done seated.
- Sit on the edge of the chair.
- Inhale, twisting torso to the left.
- Simultaneously turn the legs so that the knees point towards the left.
- Extend the right leg fully behind, while the left remains

bent at the knee in front.

- Place left hand on left knee.
- Raise your right hand, keeping it straight and looking at the fingers.
- Breathe continuously throughout.
- Hold the pose for a few seconds.
- Release to return to starting position.
- Repeat for the other side.

How it works

- Tones the pelvic region powerfully.
- Tones all the major systems along the spine, including our heart and circulatory system, to boost transport of crucial repairing, healing materials all over the body.

Other benefits

- Shapes hips.
- Trims thighs.
- Strengthens hands.
- Builds mental stamina.

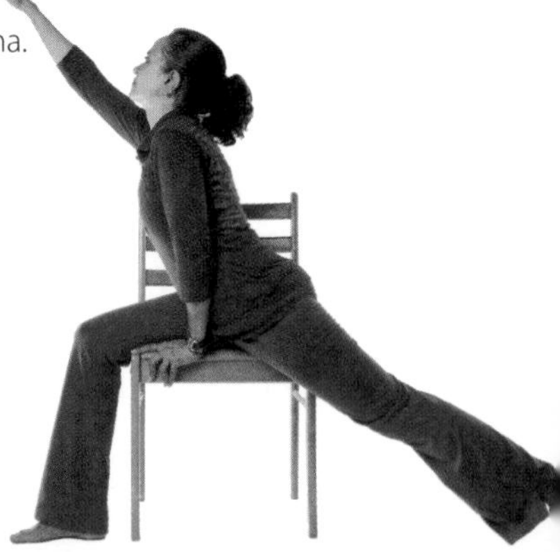

VAJROLI MUDRA (THUNDERBOLT LOCK)

Method

- Sit on a chair, with knees slightly apart.
- Shut your eyes, hands resting lightly on knees. Lean slightly forward.
- Hold your hands in the pran mudra (Page 164).
- Inhale. Draw the urinary muscles in, as you would if trying to stop urination.
- Hold the muscles for a few seconds. You may hold your breath also.
- Exhale, release the muscles.
- Repeat this a few times.

Points to note

- Avoid this practice if having any anal fissures or urinary tract infection.
- It is also a stimulating practice, so don't do it if feeling agitated or angry.

How it works

- Tones pelvic floor.
- Is preventive in prostate troubles for men.

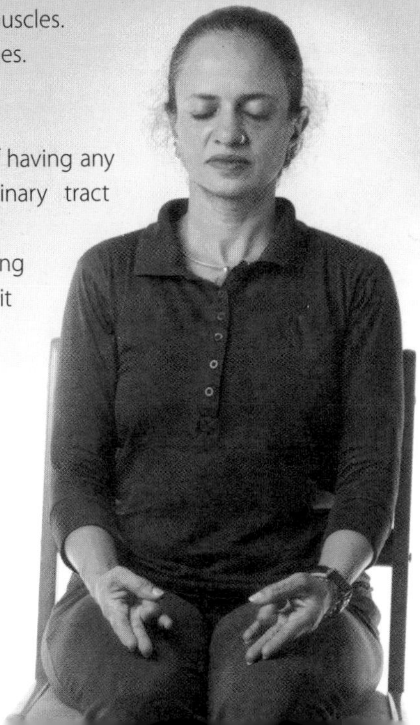

- Tightens slack vaginal muscles for women (especially after child birth); is a preventive and therapeutic in uterus prolapse.
- Therapeutic in all sexual problems, including impotence, infertility, erectile dysfunction or premature ejaculation (for men).

Other benefits

- Is a mood elevator.

PRAN MUDRA (LIFE FORCE HAND GESTURE)

Method

- To be done seated.
- Shut your eyes.
- Touch tips of the little finger and ring finger to tip of the thumb. Do for each hand.
- Hold for three to five minutes.

Points to note

Avoid when feeling very sluggish.

How it works

- It is based on the ayurvedic concept of doshas, increasing the water and earth element in the body, thus cooling and grounding us.
- Biologically, yogic hand gestures use the principle of the homunculus man or the brain representation of

our body parts, where our fingers get an amazingly disproportionate representation in our brain. By working the fingers, the nerve representations of body parts or systems is tweaked, leading to healing.

Other benefits

- Improves overall health.
- Removes tiredness.
- De-stresses.
- Cools the body, being therapeutic in inflammatory conditions.
- Prevents dry hair, skin.
- Relieves constipation.

What else?

- Sitting for long periods of time also means flabby hips. Apart from looking ungainly, this also implies weak hip bones, with the possibility of hip fractures. These poses will **prevent such hip problems**.
- Being seated in one place encourages the blood to pool at the feet. Considering that

the most important organs of our body, apart from the brain, are all in the torso, it is essential we regularly work it out. Do these yogic torso tilts to **revive all your major body systems** — digestive, circulatory, endocrine, respiratory — back to health.

- Since the uro-genital system is closely linked to our emotional upheavals, working it out also elevates our moods and **induces a powerful state of harmony**.

For real pros, work is life. At least, we spend most of our lives working. So let's check out how our love for work affects so many departments of our lives, including our looks!

The evidence is conclusive — long hours at the office can indeed damage our looks. So too the other 'so called' associated incentives like travel, hotel stay, hotel food, air-conditioning, artificial lighting, and constant exposure to electromagnetic radiation from gadgets and computers.

To look at this in greater detail, here are some hard, unsavoury facts:

- Dry eyes, usually associated with natural ageing and menopause, are now common amongst youth due to the constant exposure to dry heat caused by air-conditioning. Earlier, gritty eyes meant illness and old age. Now it just symbolises a fast-ageing pro!

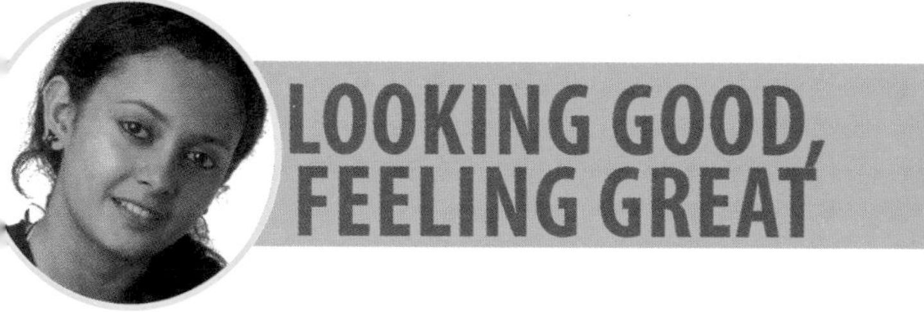

- Our protective skin can respond naturally to any adverse condition. Air-conditioning dries up the skin. Only when the skin is allowed naturally to retain moisture does it look young. So, the first effect of long hours in a centrally air-conditioned office is dry skin, with its natural, anti-ageing capacity challenged severely.

- Unfortunately, our skin's problems do not quite end there. When overexposed to the drying effect of air-conditioning, the skin may overproduce oil, causing skin eruptions. Or, if you try to beat the drying effect by moisturising constantly, the over-moisturising may end up clogging the pores. Seems skin care is not as easy as it is made out to be in cosmetic advertisements!
- Apart from clogging, an overproduction of oil could mean that your skin is readying to play host to more than 2,000 different types of germs that have been residing in your keyboard monitor, telephone handstand and desk! Not to forget the famous office-lore that 'There are hundred times more germs on your computer mouse than the toilet seat in your office loo'! And though we are natural hosts to many germs, it is when our immunity is low, or we eat food indifferently, that we become susceptible to an attack — boils, acne, rashes, fungus attacks can be signs of such breakdown in natural defences.
- Sadly all this damage does not stop with the skin. The ageing effect of a sedentary office lifestyle goes deep down, right down to your DNA. Research has established that a sedentary lifestyle shortens the biological marker for ageing, called leukocyte

telomeres. The difference could mean that just being sedentary can age you by almost a decade!

- Use of chemicals (like tricholoethylene, benezene and formaldehyde) in printing inks, detergents, varnishes, adhesives, insulation and office furniture also has its ill-effects and is commonly known to affect your bone marrow (which produces blood cells and thereby can affect your skin tone and colour), cause anaemia (iron deficiency, again needed for skin's health) and set off inflammations and various skin problems.
- Interestingly, it has been found that even if you work-out daily your gains in terms of health may be limited if the rest of your day is spent in a sedentary fashion. Muscles need constant movement to remain healthy, toned and young.
- Postural damage from a desk-bound job or bad ergonomics is also inevitable. A slump also causes an ugly double chin when the spinal curve goes out of shape. The dowager's hump — the unsightly curve on the upper back — is another deformation common amongst those who regularly slouch or respond to stress by caving in their chest. A pot belly is another of the most visible symptoms of postural mismanagement. Stress can cause localised fat deposits that lead to those ungainly abdominal tyres and love handles.
- Lack of sunlight, from being cooped up inside offices

or cars, can lead to bone loss, causing the skeletal mass to shrink. The muscle and tissue wrapped around the bones feel this impact acutely. The skin and rest of the tissue supporting it from underneath becomes loose, causing ugly folds and wrinkles. While this may make you inclined towards botox, collagen shots or silicon implants, the unnatural look this gives most people is quite a giveaway.

Now that we have proved that there is enough cause to panic if your work-style is largely sedentary, we will also present you with the solution.

For dry skin and red eyes

Yogic forward bends increase blood flow to the skin and face: the skin's moisture-retaining capacity is enhanced, its repairing mechanism is rebooted due to increased availability of blood oxygen; waste products are removed faster, preventing those pouches (under skin, on cheeks and around mouth). Blood circulation to the eyes restarts the tear mechanism so your eyes enjoy natural lubrication.

For postural deformity

Yogic stretches work by gently realigning the spine, ironing out the abuse that has been heaped on this important load-bearer of our body.

For bone loss

When muscle tone improves, the bone immediately adjoining the worked out muscle feels its positive impact. Bones need a constant supply of blood, oxygen and exercise as is provided by yogic body-toners.

For muscle tone

Unlike most other forms of exercise, yogic toners work even on the subtle muscle mass called faschia. This ensures the workout is not superficial but reaches the entire limb. So instead of the hard, steroidal look that results from other types of workouts, in yoga, the muscle gets to retain its natural supple look.

For immunity

Yogic chest openers power the immune gland, preventing you from all sorts of infections, including the ongoing assault on your skin. Improved nutrient absorption adds to this inner arsenal.

For de-stress

Yoga is a powerful de-stresser. Simply put, stress ages and ages you very fast. Other exercise forms work by creating a semblance of stress within the body. For example, in aggressive sports and exercise forms, the muscle injures itself first and as it scars it creates the tissue that gives you the tone. In yoga, this harmful stage of muscle-toning is completely by-passed. On the contrary, any stress that is part and parcel of daily life is defused through its stretches.

Some beautiful people who use yoga as part of their cosmetic ritual are David Beckham, Victoria Beckham, Rekha, Kareena Kapoor, Shilpa Shetty, Tobey Maguire, Richard Gere, Ricky Martin, Madonna, to name a few. The list, even as I write it, continues to grow longer.

International yoga has acquired a new face-lift with the yoga facial.

This niche yoga was marketed earlier as yo-tox (short for yoga plus botox) and yoga face-lift. Indian actor Shilpa Shetty glowed after giving it a try. Purists, however, like celeb yoga guru Rodney Yee, dismissed it as a scam. Modern yoga reinvents itself ever so often, finding takers amongst those who cannot invest time in classic yoga asanas.

The main benefits of these new-found yoga forms are in their compactness. They are very practical. They may be attempted anywhere without attracting curious glances, thus becoming a big hit with busy people. They activate actual acupressure points and energy meridians which lead to overall repairing and rejuvenations.

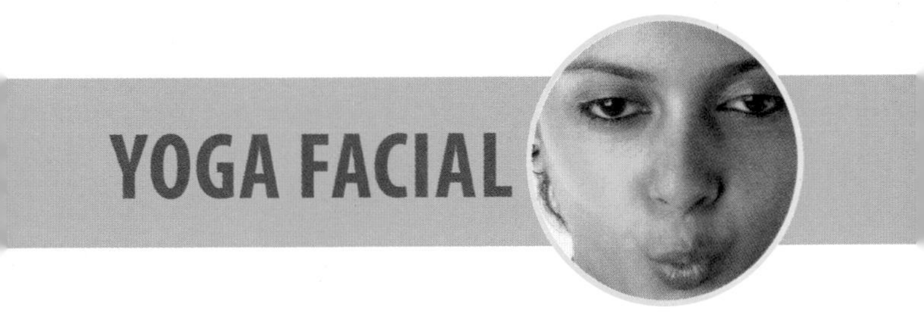

YOGA FACIAL

The crucial acupressure points that are massaged are also powerfully anti-ageing. They work on removing wrinkles and subtle tone, delicate muscles that are often neglected. They bring back elasticity to the blood vessels, so the repairing, nourishing blood flows freely back to these delicate, vulnerable spots that show ageing first. They also encourage waste removal, which otherwise shows up as puffiness. Another important point is that, unlike other facial massages which, if done wrongly, can aggravate existing flaws, these are harmless since they do not apply aggressive pressure on the face.

As a serious yoga practitioner attached to her mat, I must admit that a person who does dedicated classical yoga has no need for these gentle poses since the anti-ageing effect is naturally in-built in each classical asana. Having said that, I must say this set is perfect for those who are rushed for time but would still like a natural yoga face-lift.

VEERASANA (HERO'S POSE, ALSO REFERRED TO AS PHILOSOPHER'S POSE)

Method

- May be done seated, though proves more beneficial when done lying on the stomach (due to increased pressure from gravity).

- Cup chin with both palms, so base of hands touch lightly, while tips of fingers are touching ears.
- Place elbows on a table in front, for added pressure. Ensure inner wrists are touching.
- Shut your eyes.
- Press upper set of teeth against lower set (as if biting something), to increase pressure.
- Hold initially for thirty counts or seconds. Release.
- With regular practice, increase duration in final pose to one minute.

How it works

- The acupressure points for the lymph glands lie on the inner wrists. When a gentle pressure is maintained here, lymphatic drainage or disposal of waste is assured.
- Also, there are several acu-points along the jaw that are youth-giving. Point 35 (an inch off the ear tip) energises the entire face.
- A little away from this, slightly off the jawline, is Point 36, which fights wrinkles all over the face.
- Close beside that is Point 37, which clears wrinkles specifically from the chin area.
- Below the lip, centre of chin, is another anti-wrinkle point (Point 38), which fights facial tension.

Other benefits

- Alleviates stress.
- Point 38 is also an anti-constipation point, ensuring your gut throws out toxins that age you.

YOGA ABHASYA (YOGA PRACTICE) (LIP WORK-OUT IN THREE STEPS)

Method

- This may be done seated or standing.
- Purse your lips together, pressing them firmly, ensuring the pressure is applied right from the edge of the lips to their entire length.
- Hold with steady, firm pressure for a count of fifteen seconds initially, breathing normally.
- Release. Now move upper lip over lower lip.
- Hold for fifteen seconds.
- Release. Relax for a few moments.
- Now move lower lip over upper lip, holding for fifteen seconds.

How it works

- It activates Point 36 (mentioned above), which fights wrinkles all over the face.
- The anti-gravity drag effect works on Point 30 which lies on either side of the nose, at the edge.
- It also rejuvenates the entire face.

- Another important effect is on Point 31, the spot exactly at the centre of the upper lip.
- Apart from acu-points, the gentle workout removes crow's feet and laughter lines around the mouth and chin region, which usually reflects ageing fast.

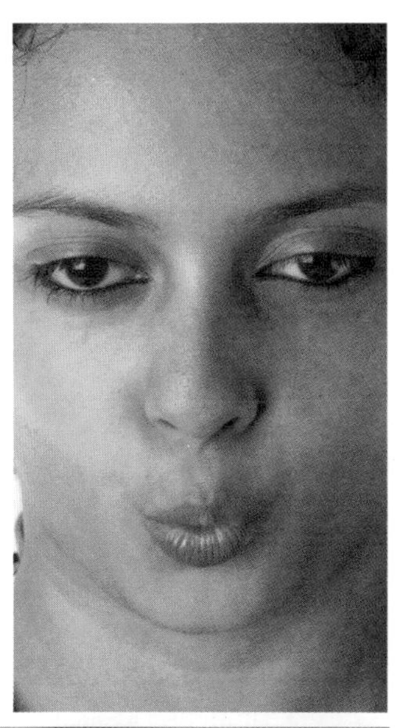

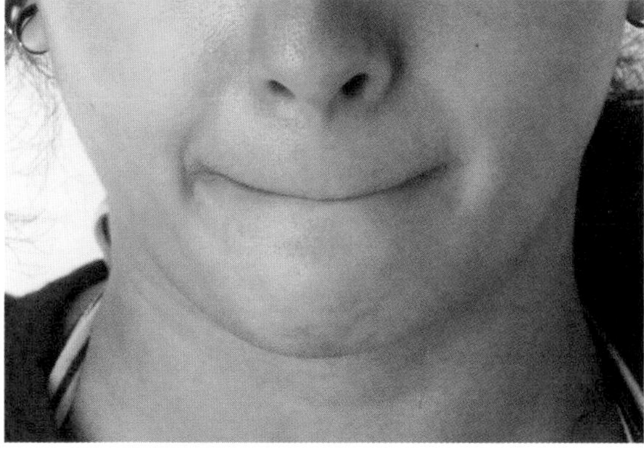

Other benefits

- Point 30 also works on sinus points, relieving congestion.
- Point 31 is an emergency relief point that has a powerful impact on the pituitary or the master gland. This affects the hormones of the entire body. The effect is powerful for all major organ systems.
- This also affects our emotions positively.

SUKU PRANAYAMA (HAPPY BREATHING PRACTICE)

Method

- May be done seated or standing.
- Purse your lips to form an 'O'.
- Inhale deeply, so the cheeks cave in.
- Shut your mouth, pressing lips back to normal.
- Exhale from the nostril.
- This is one round. You may do up to nine rounds.

Points to note

- Please note that since this involves mouth breathing, you should never attempt this practice when in a polluted, dusty place or where the quality of air is suspect since that could lead to respiratory problems.
- This is a simpler version of the anti-ageing cooling breathing practices called sheetali (cooling) or sheetkari (whistling).
- To be avoided by those clinically depressed.

- To be avoided by those with extreme low blood pressure.
- Avoid when having congestion or cold.

How it works

- It is a powerful anti-ageing practice, since it tweaks the parasympathetic nervous system, needed for repair and rejuvenation.
- Apart from that, it also works out the cheeks and the delicate region around the mouth, preventing sagging and removing fine laughter lines.
- Reduces inner inflammation, which causes oxidative stress that results in ageing.

Other benefits

- This is said to impact hunger centres in your brain, controlling emotional bingeing.
- It is a cooling practice which is an immediate de-stresser.
- Lowers blood pressure.
- Lowers fever. May be used in hot climate to cool down.

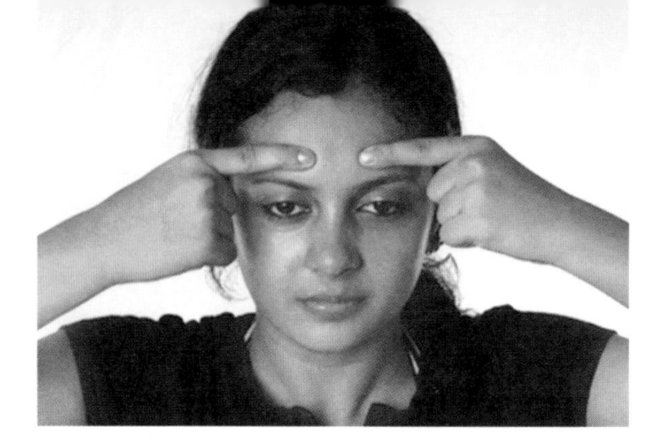

KAPALARANDRA DHAUTI (SKULL-CLEANSING MOVES)

Method

- May be done seated or standing.
- Use index finger to apply the soft pressure required in this exercise.
- Shut eyes. Start this practice with your right eye.
- Lightly tap the entire socket of the eye with your index finger.
- Do five times for each eye.
- Keep eyes shut for a while before opening.

Points to note

- The movement must start from where the eyebrow begins. Then move outwards, towards the temple.
- The touch should be a light and gentle tap.
- In any facial exercise, especially around the delicate areas, the skin should never be stretched.

- It may even be done several times during the day for stress relief.

How it works

- The eye socket region has major acu-points that deal with overall health and which are believed to be anti-ageing.
- These points also relieve tension, which can mar good looks!
- They are therapeutic in eye strain, they help clear vision and dry eye syndrome by promoting blood circulation.
- They gently prevent the skin from drooping at this area.

YOGA ABHASYA (YOGA PRACTICE) (CHEEK WORKOUT)

Method

- May be done seated or standing.
- Puff out cheeks as much as you can, filling it with air.
- Ensure the inside of the lips is also similarly puffed up.
- Then place your index fingers on either cheek, applying a light pressure, causing a resistance against the puffed cheeks.
- Hold for fifteen seconds.
- Release. Repeat a few times.

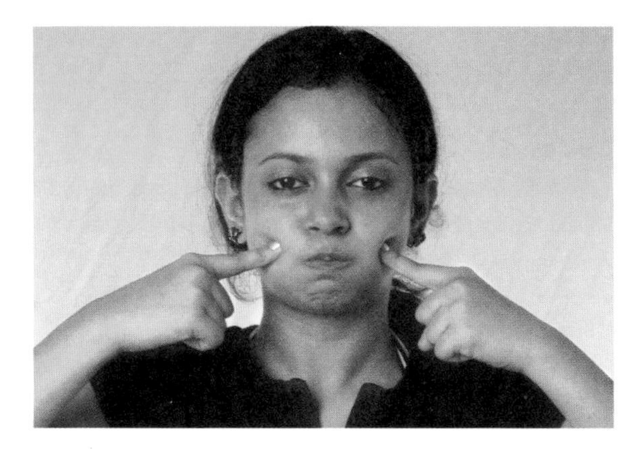

Points to note

To enhance the benefits, when the face is held in the final position, you may splash some cold water on the puffed cheeks and face.

How it works

- This works out the muscles in the cheeks, preventing sagging.
- It is a powerful energiser.
- Acu-points worked out include Point 32 (or face tonic point, said to tone up the entire face); Point 30 (sinus relief and facial repair); Point 29 (tip of nose, cures addictive behaviour and nasal congestion), needed to maintain face glow; Point 31 (emergency relief and master gland control); and Point 36 (fights wrinkles on face).

Other benefits

- Works out Point 28 (an inch above, on the nose bridge). This works on nutrient absorption needed to maximise youthfulness, health and emotional stamina.
- Also works on psychosomatic points, like those which control addictive behaviour.
- The master gland is tweaked, in turn having a powerful effect on hormonal flow, metabolic health and emotional harmony.
- The nasal and sinus points massaged boost respiratory capacity.

Points to note

If you do not have epilepsy, heart problems or blood pressure, you can hold your breath for a count of four to ten in the final stage.

What else?

- They are all cure-all practices, not just keeping you good-looking and youthful but **preventing a whole cluster of ailments.**
- They **deepen respiratory capacity** by clearing congestion and opening respiratory channels through the acu-points activated in the sinus cavities inside the skull.
- Most also **work on metabolism**, indirectly helping with weight loss goals.
- They rid the face and neck region of stress-related stiffness, **making you feel lighter** and more in control.

Looks are important, but what really matters at the end of the day is correct posture. Yet, we spend more time and money on the former. A laidback lifestyle, including sitting or standing for a long time in one position, ruins the posture by making the stomach sag, the spine cave in, the upper body hunch, and legs misaligned. A spine comes with inbuilt weaknesses — it has curves which can either help hold the body against gravity or collapse awkwardly when we slump too much.

Disuse of muscles that support the posture can destroy the subtle nerve-brain-muscle communication. This communication has to be in peak condition to maintain right posture. When this communication collapses, we end up using wrong muscles for daily chores, further affecting the elegance of our posture.

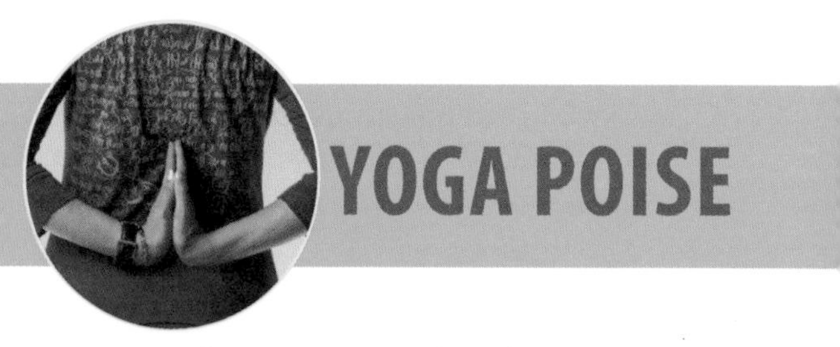

Intriguingly, even stress can hurt the primary control region of our body. This region lies at the upper back and neck region where the skull (which along with the brain weighs up to an impressive six kilograms) rests on the spine (on the vertebra rightly called the Atlas). Stress ruins one's posture by tensing the muscles, shortening the fibres, creating stiffness. Only when muscles are elastic and supple can our body call upon its shock-absorbing capacity that helps it endure the pressure of daily movements and actions. The hugely popular and effective science of the Alexander techniques which use postural corrections to transform life, is based on the belief that even communication and voice throw is linked intimately with our posture.

It is believed that every twenty minutes our body requires a shift from the posture it is holding (we even change sides while sleeping due to this basic biological need). When this does not happen, our muscles start losing tone. Recent research shows even people who have a daily exercise regime of an hour do not benefit from their workouts much if the rest of their day is confined to one posture. Our musculo-skeletal system needs constant movement to maintain its tone. That means we need to factor in stretch breaks throughout the day to maintain a youthful spine.

Try these stretches to iron out postural distortions.

DWIKONASANA (DOUBLE-ANGLE STRETCH)

Method

- May be done seated or standing.
- If doing seated, ensure you are sitting on the edge of a chair.
- Spread legs.
- If you are doing it standing, then spread legs wide apart. Feet pointed straight.
- Clasp hands behind your back, fingers interlocked.
- Stretch arms out fully behind you.
- Inhale. Exhaling, bend down, but keep the arms still stretched out behind.
- Bend forehead between legs, or place forehead on the chair's edge, or between the knees.
- Continue breathing normally, holding the stretch.
- Release. Repeat a few times.

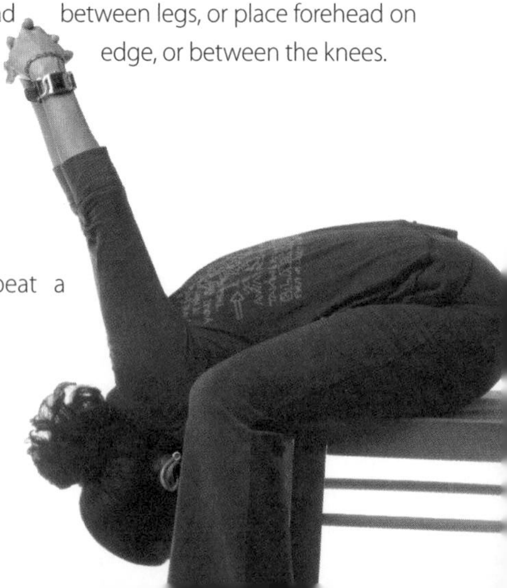

Points to note

- You can keep pushing the arms, depending on flexibility. If you're a beginner, don't push too hard. The ability to keep the arms up is a matter of regular practice.
- Avoid this pose or bend lightly if suffering from severe lower backache.

How it works

- Gives the back a powerful stretch.
- Works on the muscles supporting posture.

Other benefits

- Expands the chest, giving emotional uplift.
- Boosts respiratory capacity.
- Hikes metabolism.
- Stimulates mentally.
- Trims arms; and if done standing, also tones legs.

SAMKONASANA (RIGHT ANGLE POSE)

Method

- Done seated.
- Move chair slightly away from the desk, keeping it at arm's length.
- Sit on the chair.
- Inhale, raising arms overhead. Cup either elbow.

- Exhaling, bend forehead, placing elbows on the table, with head hanging between hands. Rest forehead on the table edge.
- Hold the pose, feeling the gush of blood in the head, face and lips.
- Breathe normally. Relax, return to starting position.

How it works

- Gives a powerful traction to the spine.
- Is excellent in treating upper body stiffness, neck pain and aches.

Other benefits

- Cools your mind with a rush of blood.
- De-stresses, irons out anger and other negativities.
- Keeps face young and fresh, eyes sparkling, promotes hair growth.
- Is therapeutic in blood pressure problems and diabetes.

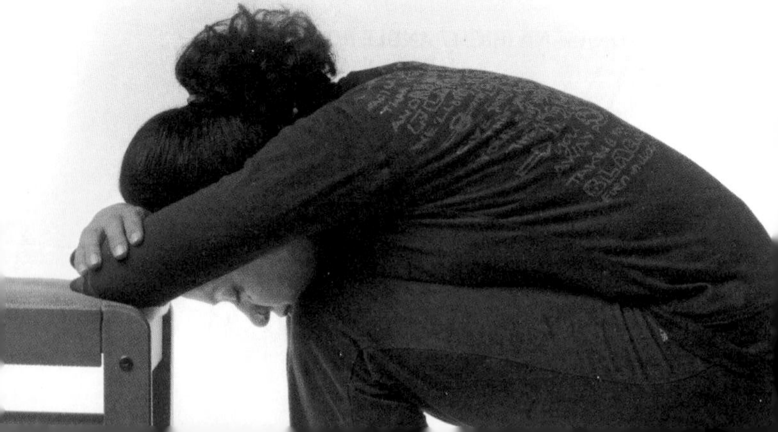

PRANAMASANA (PRAYER POSE, HANDS BEHIND)

Method

- May be done standing or seated.
- Inhale, passing your hands behind.
- Exhale, bringing palms together. Essentially, you must make a namaste/prayer gesture behind you.
- Continue normal breathing.
- Hold for as long as is comfortable.
- Release. Repeat a few times.

Points to note

- Those with very stiff bodies may not be able to bring their hands together, particularly at the base. But regular practice will rectify this.
- Some with faulty nerve-limb co-ordination may not be able to even get the palms to touch. Such practitioners may just lock fingers initially to facilitate neuro-muscular training.
- Those who can perform this pose with ease

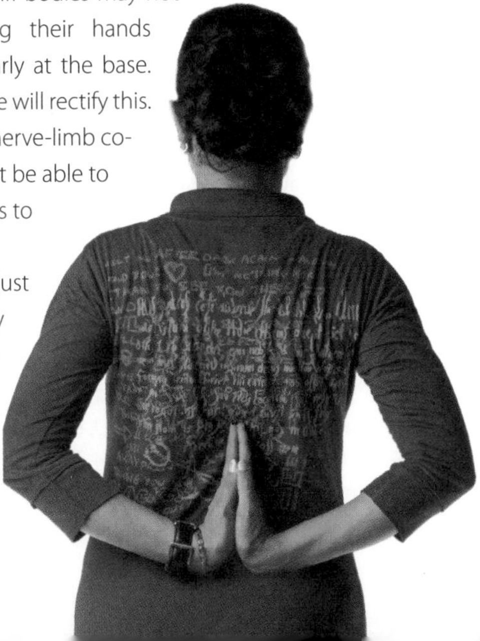

can enhance benefits by moving the hands higher up, so it is between the shoulder blades. This deepens the stretch and opens up the chest wider.

How it works

- It is a gentle, but powerful rectifier of spinal defects.
- It opens up the soft muscle tissue, the suppleness of which is crucial for spinal health.

Other benefits

- It is a very safe practice, encouraged as therapy in most major ailments.
- Is a chest-opener, and enhances breathing.
- For the above reason, is a mood elevator.

GOMUKASANA (COW-FACE POSE)

Method

- May be done seated or standing.
- Inhale. Pass right hand over the shoulder, palm facing the back.
- Simultaneously pass left hand behind, to grasp right hand.
- Exhale. Hook fingers.
- Hold for a few seconds, with normal breathing.
- Keep face straight, back erect, avoiding the tendency to tilt.
- Relax and hold the pose. Repeat for the other side.

- After regular practice, hold longer in final pose.

Points to note

Some beginners may find they are unable to make contact between both hands on the less favoured side. For example, right-handers may have difficulty on the left side, and vice-versa. Hold a kerchief or scarf between the hands initially. With regular practice this misalignment is soon rectified. Usually, it can be achieved even in four to six weeks.

How it works

- Is therapeutic in most spinal ailments.
- Is used to treat body stiffness arising from degenerative problems like blood pressure, diabetes and obesity.
- It rectifies misalignment of the spine and rest of the body.

Other benefits

- Opens the chest, boosting respiratory capacity.
- Uplifts emotionally.

ARDHA CHANDRASANA (CRESCENT, WITH SUPPORT)

Method

- Done standing. Stand at arm's length from the desk.
- Place left hand on the desk. Inhale.
- Exhale, tilt towards the left.
- Inhale. Exhaling, lift right leg straight up and out in the air, as high as you can.
- Hold, breathing normally.
- Exhale, drop leg back down.
- Repeat for the left side.

Points to note

You may do thrice for each leg. Or hold for a long time for each leg. The latter is an advanced practice, since you need muscular stamina to hold a pose for longer duration.

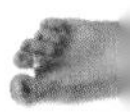

How it works

- Strengthens the legs, teaching it to take the load off the spine and the knees.
- It works out the spine and spinal nerves.
- Is therapeutic in all spinal problems, from lower back to upper back. Also a preventive in all spinal ailments.
- Improves balance, also involved intimately with posture.

Other benefits

- Harmonises both brain hemispheres, bringing mental equilibrium.
- Inculcates a sense of fun and lightness of spirit.
- Used in therapy in other ailments related to the uro-genital system (tones the pelvic region), the knees and the digestive tract.
- Enhances memory and mental focus, due to the impact on the cerebellum and the balancing mechanism in the brain.

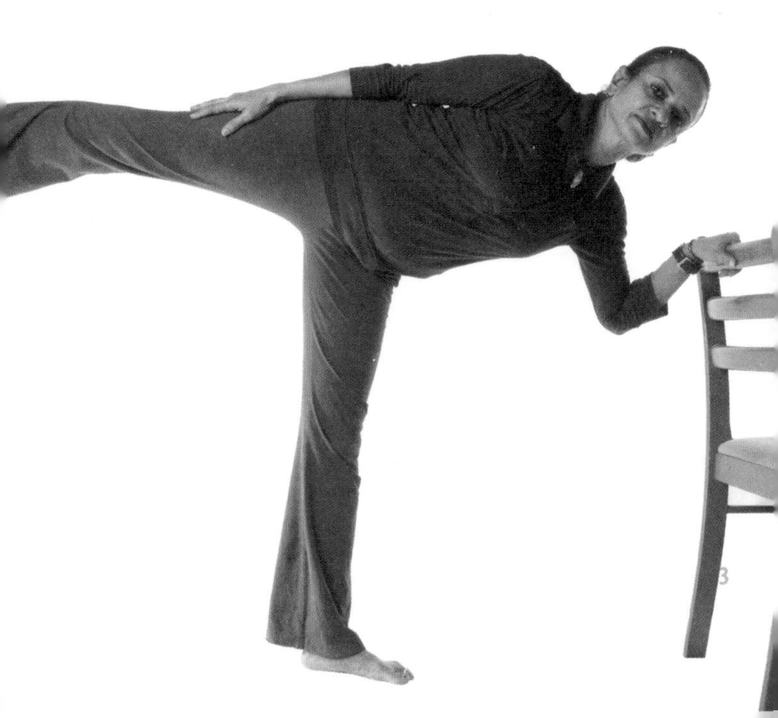

What else?

- Not many people know that neck and shoulder muscles are involved with efficient respiration. So, most hard-working people not only compromise their posture but ruin their breathing too. Use the above poses not only to tone up your neck and shoulders, but also to **breathe easy**!
- All poses are preventive and **therapeutic in neck pain**, which has reached epidemic proportions amongst office-goers.
- All these poses also **de-stress powerfully** and elevate you emotionally.

All those yogic texts promising that a regular sadhana will make you glow like 'kama deva' — the god of love — simply mean that yoga will keep you age-less and youthful! Myths of yogic greats like Babaji (a Chiranjeevi or the eternal one who, legend has it, still roams in the Himalayan wilds) enthral serious yoga practitioners, partly because it is also believed that Babaji, though hundreds of years old, still glows with the youthfulness of a twenty-year-old! In fact, the yogic text of Hatha yoga pradipika by Swami Swatmarama assures us that not only will we glow, but also smell fragrant through regular sadhana or yogic practice!

That is not so tough to accept, scientifically. Except where the problems are hereditary (like genetic baldness or greying), it is now medically validated that lush hair growth and a glowing skin depend largely on one's lifestyle,

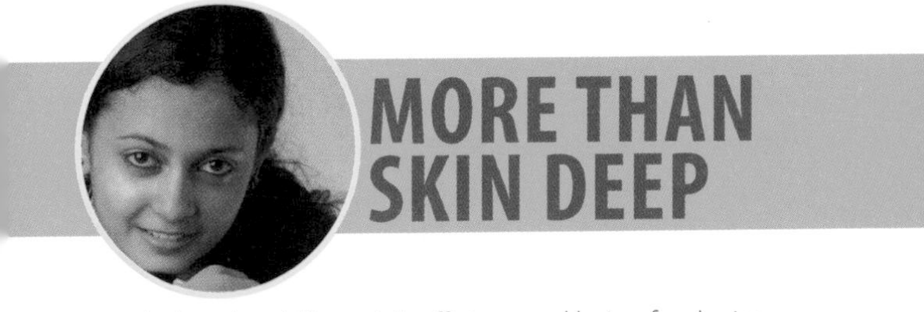

MORE THAN SKIN DEEP

including the ability to lob off stress and being food-wise.

Hair fall may even be caused by lack of sunlight, which helps our body produce the much-needed Vitamin D. And if your job requires you to be cooped up in the office for long or you shun sunlight entirely, you may well expect hair to show its distress. Similarly, even jet lag can cause delayed hair fall — some triggers for frequent-long-haul fliers include excessive dehydration (from air-conditioning), sudden climatic changes and strange foods. Dehydration also hits the skin's moisture-retaining capacity, causing the puffed under-eye look (from lack of blood circulation which selectively deposits fat underneath or delays removal of toxins), dry or wrinkled skin, etc.

A mismanaged diet can compound all this. Lack of iron, zinc (needed also to heal wounds), a sluggish liver, excessive consumption of caffeine, sugar (read bottled drinks), and low protein intake can ruin hair and skin tone. Hormonal upsets, several medications, including some we take for treatment in cardiovascular problems, joint pains, hormonal imbalances or stress relief, also affect our skin and hair health. Popping pills to control acidity can draw from our scarce nutrient stores. The cluster of lifestyle-provoked ailments, like metabolic syndrome, adult onset diabetes and arthritis, also affect hair and skin health. Diabetes and magnesium absorption capacity are linked. And magnesium is seriously needed in our body to fight oxidative stress that ages us.

The major culprit is, of course, stress, because it creates a negative hormonal loop. The body, when it is in this state of emergency, directs all its resources to those parts that require immediate attention, like skin and hair.

Where does yoga come into all these lifestyle issues?

- It is the most effective stress-buster. It nullifies the deadly residue of stress (free radical damage) that causes ageing.
- It spikes metabolic efficiency, meaning where earlier the body rejected nutrients, it now begins to absorb and store them.
- It detoxifies the liver back to efficiency — a super-efficient liver is an absolute must for skin-hair health because it encourages the enzymatic reactions that assure it.
- Most significantly, it sends a powerful gush of blood to the scalp and face region. The tone of the vessels that supply to these regions is also improved. All micro-vessels, nerves, muscles that service this region — which have been neglected for the most part — are completely rejuvenated back to youthful fitness.
- Equally, significant marmic points or acupressure points, through which major energy meridians run, are tweaked. The face and neck region are also a major thoroughfare for these energy channels.

Increasing amounts of evidence continues to pile up on the yoga–youth connection. But those who practice do not need to wait for such evidence: for them, the mirror speaks the truth! This explains why yoga is such a hot favourite with celebrities for whom looking good is very important.

To get that yogic glow, try these classical anti-ageing poses.

PASCHIMOTTANSANA (FORWARD BEND)

Method

- Sit on a chair.
- Inhale, raising hands overhead.
- Exhaling, raise both legs up, as high as you can. You may use the table for support, on which to place your legs.
- Simultaneously, reach out both your hands towards your toes.
- Drop head towards thighs gently.

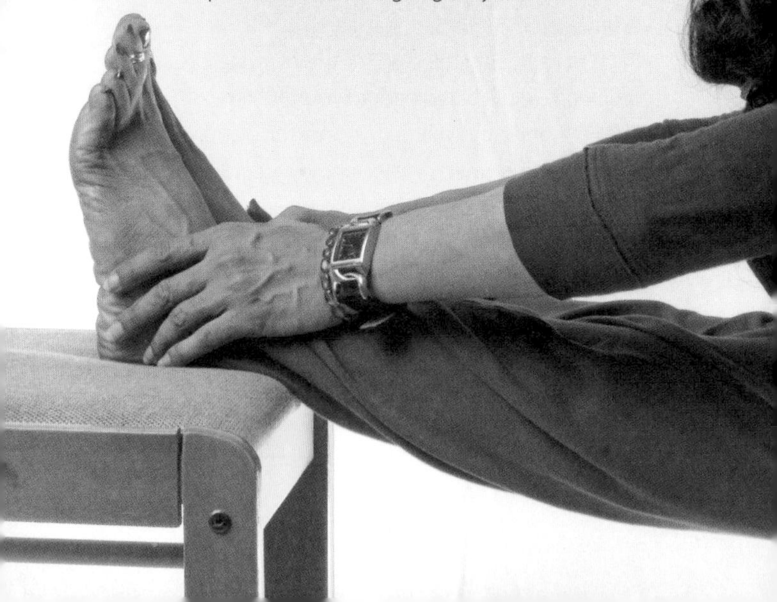

- Clasp hands around thighs to hold the legs up and head down.
- Hold the pose for as long as you can, breathing normally.
- Release. Repeat a few times.

Points to note

- Initially, beginners will not be able to raise both legs up very high. Do whatever is in your capacity.

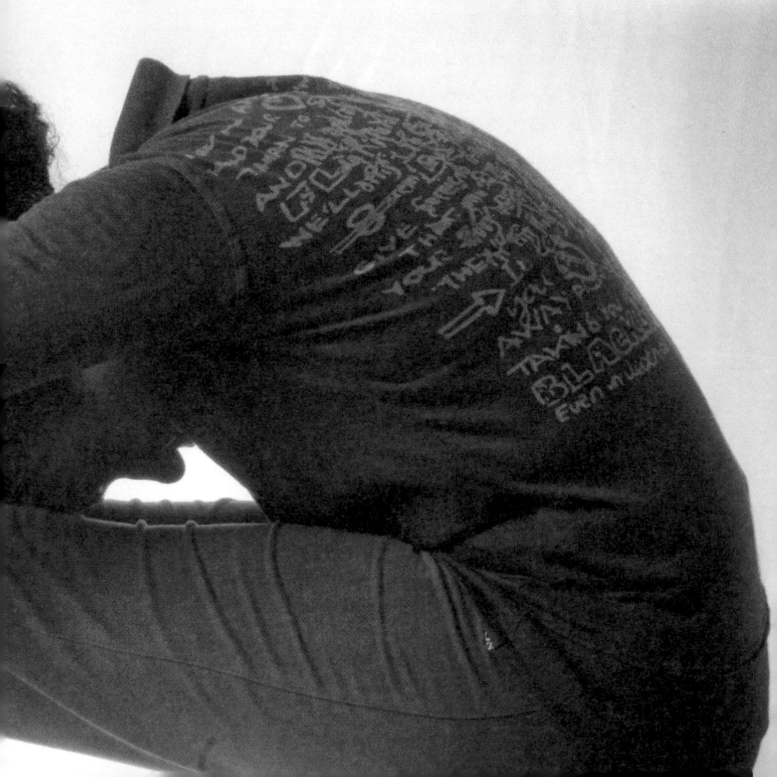

- Place legs well on the chair seat, otherwise it may be difficult to hold the pose.
- Use a low stool on which to rest legs, instead of raising them, in case of spinal problems.
- Avoid this pose in case of acute lower back problems and high blood pressure or cardiac problems.

How it works

- The gush of blood to the face and neck improves circulation to the facial skin and scalp.
- It is curative in most skin ailments, including chronic problems like dry skin, acne, etc.
- The pressure on the gut helps improve digestion, metabolism and nutrient absorption.
- Is a powerful stress-buster.

Other benefits

- Helps relieve knee pain.
- Is preventive in spinal disorders.
- Aids weight loss.
- Tones limbs.
- Is therapeutic in digestive problems.
- Controls diabetes.

PADAHASTASANA (FORWARD BEND, HAND-TO-FOOT POSE)

- Done seated.
- Sit on the edge of the chair. (May also be done standing to make it more effective.
- Inhale.
- Exhaling, bend gently, lowering head down and placing the forehead between legs on the chair edge.
- You can also dangle it beyond the edge of the chair, between the knees.
- Hang the hands loose, or hold ankles lightly.
- Breathe evenly. Inhaling, return gently back to sitting position.

Points to note

- Avoid in case of acute lower backache and high blood pressure.
- When lifting head and torso back to the starting position, always come up very slowly. Otherwise you may feel

dizzy. It is also more effective that way, in terms of building the tone of blood vessels.

How it works

Same as above.

Other benefits

- Gives a definitive traction to the spine.
- Blood gushes to the head, cooling it, especially when stressed out or angry. Aids in anger and anxiety control.
- Is therapeutic in respiratory problems.
- Preventive and therapeutic in upper-body aches.
- Relieves headaches.

VATA NAASHAK (HAND GESTURE TO CONTROL THE WIND ELEMENT)

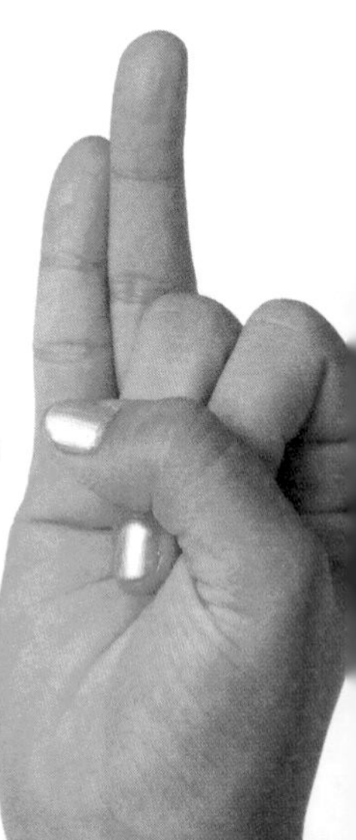

Method

- Sit with spine erect.
- Ideally shut eyes since mudras are best done in a meditative manner.
- Press middle and index fingers of both hands down towards base of thumb.
- Press thumb over these fingers, to hold them down.
- Hold for three to five minutes.

How it works

- Calms the mind; relieves negativities.
- It is said to boost the water element, thus therapeutic for dry, flaky skin and dry, brittle hair.

Other benefits

- Reduces symptoms of inflammation such as fever or throat.
- Relieves constipation.
- Relieves arthritic pain.

Point to note

Avoid if feeling sluggish.

PRITHVI MUDRA (HAND GESTURE TO INCREASE THE EARTH ELEMENT)

Method

- Done seated.
- Sit in a meditative fashion, eyes shut, since mudras are most effective when done meditatively.
- Touch tip of ring finger with the tip of the thumb for both hands.
- Hold for three to five minutes.

Points to note

Avoid in case of excessive kapha dosha, or congestion.

How it works

- It increases the element of earth in the body.
- Is calming.
- Is used in halting premature greying caused due to stress.
- Is therapeutic in hair fall, dry skin, brittle nails.

Other benefits

- Helps fight inflammatory conditions.
- Strengthens bones.
- Relieves hyperthyroidism.

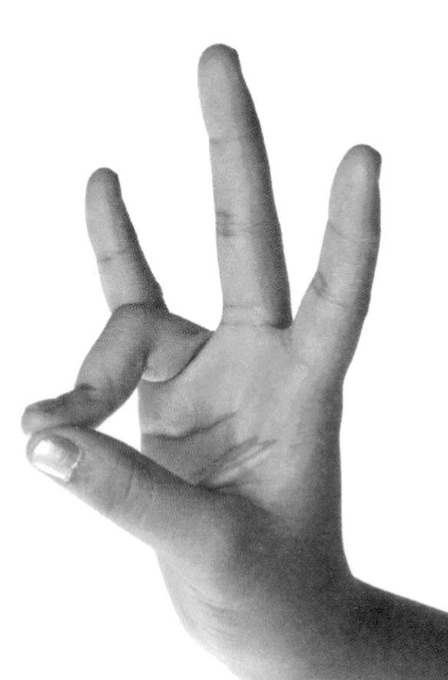

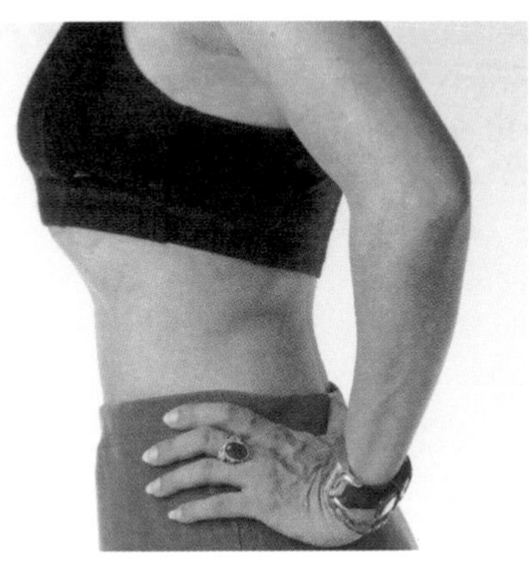

AGNISARA KRIYA (METABOLIC FIRE PRACTICE)

Method

- This may be done seated or standing. It must always be done on an empty stomach.
- Inhale and exhale a few times.
- Inhale. Exhaling forcefully, cave in stomach as much as you can.
- Hold the breath.
- Now flap the stomach muscles in and out.
- Do up to ten to fifteen flaps initially.
- This is one round. Do three rounds.

How it works

- It works out flaccid stomach muscles and the entire gut.

- Boosts metabolism and nutrient absorption.

Other benefits

- Perks up mood, is stimulating, removes lethargy.
- Helps with fat release.

Points to note

Avoid if having stomach problems, inflammatory conditions, heart and blood pressure problems. It is a cleansing practice, a precursor to pranayama or breathing practices.

What else?

- The gush of blood impacts our brain, calming it down. During stress or overwhelming anger, the blood flow is redirected to the legs. This is rectified through such poses, **cooling us emotionally**.
- The **abdomen is tightened**, removing belly fat.
- The **spine is lengthened**, so acts as a preventive and is therapeutic in spinal problems that arise from a sedentary lifestyle.
- The mudras are **therapeutic in several ailments** caused by inner inflammation and oxidative stress, being cure-all practices.

A toned body not only looks good but also conveys unstated elegance and style. If a first impression is indeed the last, then your body language — healthy and toned — must rank more than what you wear. It also subtly conveys the idea of inherent discipline because a healthy body can't be had from a bottle, or be obtained under a cosmetic surgeon's scalpel.

Hatha yoga pradipika promises that a regular yoga practice will endow you with a lean body while your skin will turn luminous. No wonder then that yoga is such a big hit with body-worshippers all around the world. Indians too are rediscovering its magic.

But a toned look is not only about looking good. Ideally, your muscle tone should be such that it helps take the load off your joints, keeping them healthier for longer. The joints get lubricated and less creaky. The connective

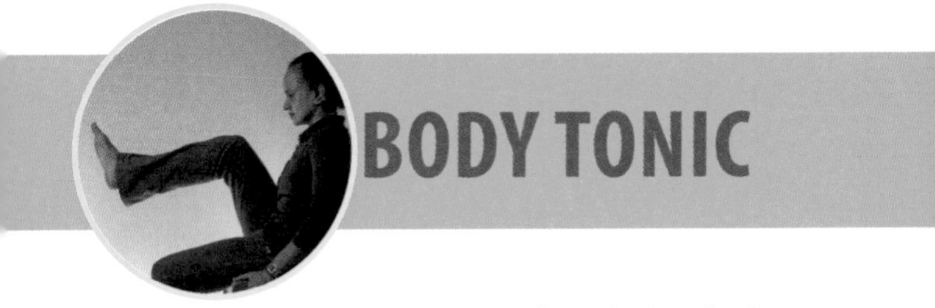

tissue, which can get chronically inflamed when badly used or when unused, becomes healthy once again. When legs are strong, they take the load off the spine (helping you retain your posture). There is less chronic fatigue.

More then this, even bones become stronger. For bones to become dense (and healthy, so they are able to store not only important minerals and nutrients but also produce more blood cells and immune cells), the muscles near them have to be strong. Workouts that challenge the muscle indirectly, but definitely, impact the bone. So both complement each other's growth and strength.

Since this sort of health comes from deep down, the body enjoys a rare youthfulness for a long time. In fact, inactivity and ageing are linked — a young but inactive person may be biologically older than a person who is only chronologically older, but more active.

So I hope by now everyone knows the secret to losing and maintaining weight: muscle tone! When your body's muscle weight is more, you burn more calories even when inactive. For those who like to collect statistics on such things, here is one: muscle burns almost three to five times more calories than the fat in your body. Also, it is metabolically more active, which means you enjoy a healthy metabolism that knows how to absorb the nutrients from all that you eat and distribute it to the sites that need it. Those who are unhealthy and lack muscle tone may eat healthily, but the body's mechanism to use the nutrients gets distorted and cranky.

So, it is tone-up time with yoga! Remember that, though exercises like walking or running power your legs, yoga stretches are the ones which work out the subtle muscle mass. Such stretches make the legs flexible as well as superbly toned.

PAWAN MUKTASANA (ENERGY-RELEASING POSE)

Method

- Stand a foot or so from a desk or some solid support.
- Bend hands, to grasp each elbow.
- Inhale.
- Exhale. Place elbows on desk, leaning forward.
- Continue normal breathing.
- Press down heels.
- Push hips out and up deliberately, feeling the stretch powerfully at the back of your legs. Hold the pose as long as you can, breathing normally throughout,

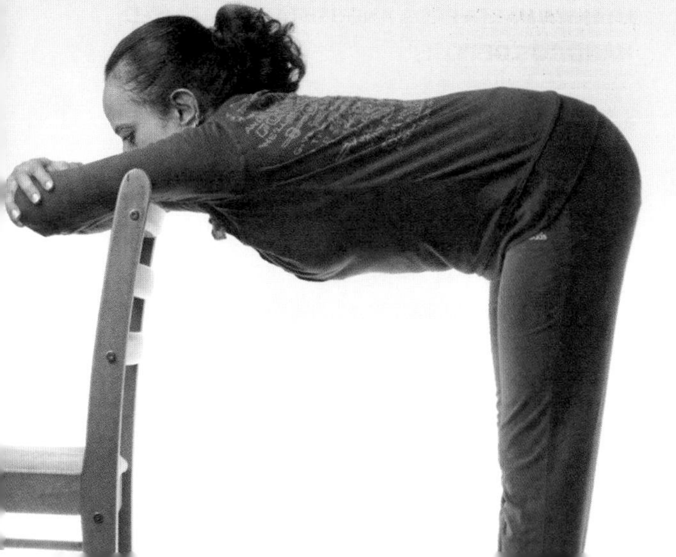

feeling the stretch extending from the soles of your feet, along the back of the legs up to your back.
- Release. You can do this several times during the day.

How it works

- It gives a powerful stretch to the spine and legs.
- Makes the legs shapely, trimming back of hips and thighs.
- Tones arms, if you learn to take weight on them.

Other benefits

- Tones spinal nerves, impacting mood positively.
- Is relaxing and rejuvenating. Removes tension along the entire back.

UTTHITA HASTA PADA ANGUSHTASANA (RAISED HAND-TO-TOE POSE)

Method

- Done standing.
- Do this with a prop, like a belt.
- Stand at an arm's distance from a support, like a desk.
- Place left arm on the support firmly.
- Fold the belt to pass it around the sole of your right foot, holding the belt ends in your right hand. Inhale. Exhaling, pull up the belt so the right leg is raised high, sideways.

- Hold for as long as you can, breathing normally.
- Release and repeat a few times.
- Relax. Then repeat the entire sequence for the other side.

How it works

- It works out the hip joints, usually a victim of a sedentary lifestyle.
- Tones legs.

Other benefits

- Improves posture.
- Boosts breathing.
- Tones the uro-genital system powerfully.

EKA PADA CHAKRASANA (ONE-LEGGED CYCLING)

Method

- Sit on a chair.
- Hold back rest for support.
- Breathe normally throughout practice.
- Raise right leg so knee is raised high, almost touching the stomach.
- Drop it, simultaneously raising the left leg. This is one round.
- Repeat up to ten-fifteen rounds.

Points to note

You may incorporate breath sequencing after a few weeks, inhaling as you raise the right leg, and exhaling while dropping it.

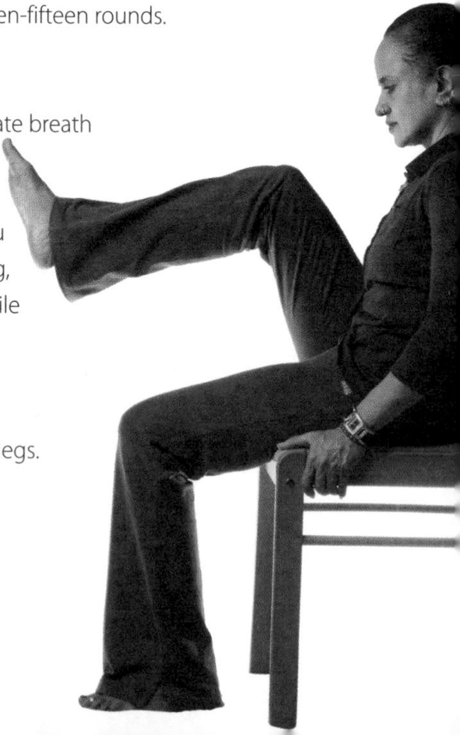

How it works

- Works out the legs.

Other benefits

- Improves blood circulation all over the body.
- Removes mental lethargy.
- Tones stomach.
- Fights flab at hips.

UTKATASANA (SQUAT POSE, WITH WALL SUPPORT)

Method

- Stand with your back against a wall, feet a foot away from the wall. Feet should ideally be together. Beginners may place them slightly apart.
- Feet must remain pointed out in front.
- Let hands hang loose by the side, or hold them out in front (the latter version serves to tone arms and build stamina).
- Inhale. Exhaling, lower hips against the wall.
- Go as low as you can.
- Hold the pose, leaning gently against the wall and breathing normally.
- Release to return to starting position.
- Repeat a few times.

Points to note

- Increase duration of the final pose with regular practice. This will enhance the toning effect.

How it works

- It aids weight loss by hiking metabolism.
- It tones the entire body, including the abdomen.

Other benefits

- A powerful spinal workout.
- Is therapeutic in most ailments.

VIRABHADRASANA (WARRIOR POSE)

Method

- Done standing.
- Stand with feet far apart. Arms must be held straight out, at shoulder-level.
- Point right foot outwards, so that it is parallel under the right arm. Left foot is slightly pointed towards the left.
- Inhale. Exhaling, lower hips lightly so the right leg is bent at the knee, while the left straightens to accommodate the squat (as shown in the image alongside).
- Hold the pose, maintaining your focus on the right hand.
- Relax from pose, returning to starting point.
- Repeat for the other side, holding for an equal length of time.
- Repeat a few times.

Points to note

Duration in the final pose must be increased for true impact.

How it works

- It tones the arms and legs by creating a muscular demand.

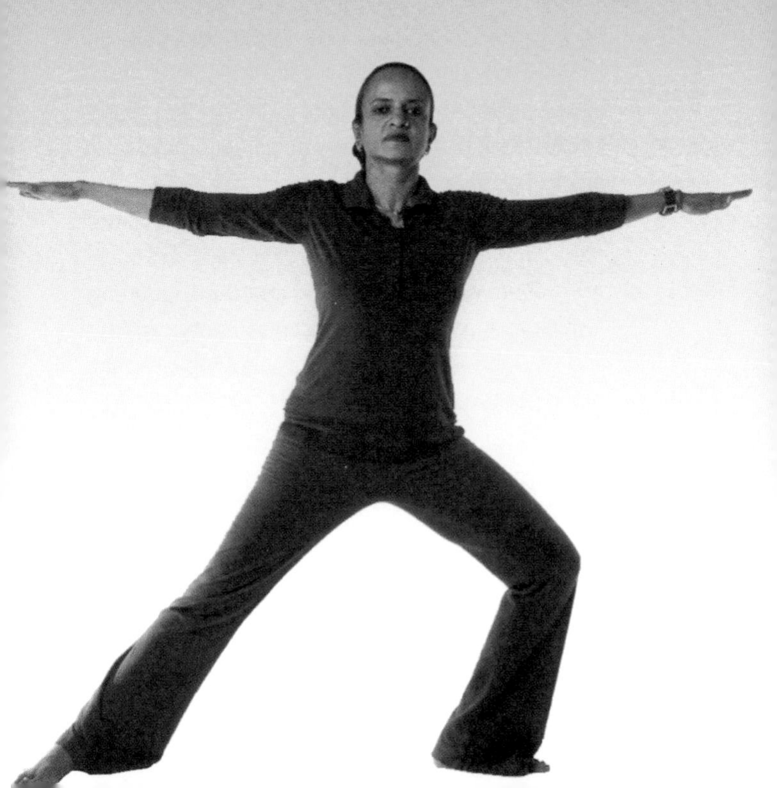

Other benefits

- Expands chest muscles and rib cage, facilitating breathing.
- This boosts mood and energy levels.
- Powers mental and physical stamina tremendously.
- Is the base position for other powerful poses and prepares you for them.

What else?

- All leg toners also **affect your mood positively**, by boosting blood circulation.
- Because of improved circulation, skin tone and health is reflected in the **yogic glow** you get through regular practice of these moves.
- All leg toners also improve **mental focus and clarity** due to improved blood supply to the heart and brain.
- Arm toners work on the chest and the supporting respiratory mechanism to **boost respiratory capacity** and efficient use of oxygen. This also impacts one's mood positively.

Belly fat is not just about mismanaged body aesthetics, it is also a pointer to hidden health disasters. This explains why abdominal tyres afflict skinny individuals — it is the first indicator of stress. Stress is what makes the body selectively deposit fat at the abdomen. Intuitive doctors use belly fat to identify the onset of cardiac problems and circulatory disasters.

Did you know that belly fat acquires a special, unwanted importance of its own? It becomes an organ in its own right, even releasing hormones which are at variance with the body's needs! This can play havoc with all our systems, ruining several departments in our cosmetic armoury — skin and hair for starters. It can set off the hunger button even when we are not hungry, thus slowly adding inches elsewhere.

Of course, belly fat also ruins silhouettes. It hits posture, making us lose inches in height faster as we gain

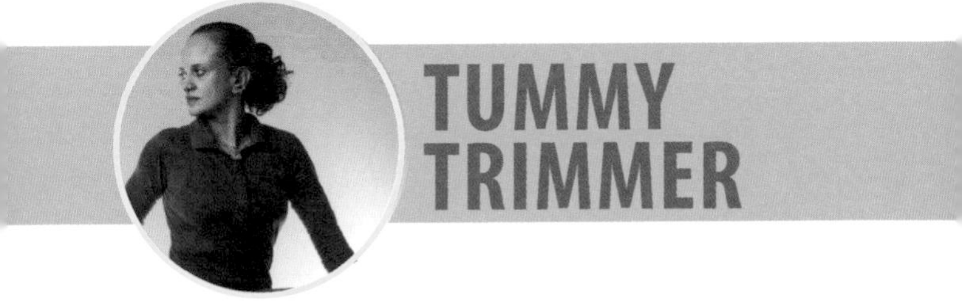

in years. It is often either the cause or effect of an ugly slump that grows into the unsightly dowager's hump on the upper back.

Your torso is also where most of your organs are stacked up. A desk-bound job makes the entire circulatory system sluggish, pooling the blood to the legs. Thus, using these yogic tummy trimmers is a good way to pump some life into the circulation at the torso, so that the digestive system becomes an efficient aide in your cosmetic repair kit. We can't forget that it is blood which reaches the repairing agents like vitamin C to the skin, and special nutrients like vitamin A to the scalp to give that luster to your hair. These simple yogic practices have a larger, hidden agenda — to give you that fabled yoga glow!

NAUKASANA (BOAT POSE, SEATED VERSION)

Method

- To be done seated in a chair.
- Sit in the middle of the chair, sideways if the chair has a backrest.
- Inhale, placing both hands on either side of the knees.
- Exhale, hoist knees up, lifting feet off the ground, so the bent legs remain raised in the air.
- Inhale, dropping feet back to the ground.
- This is one round.
- Do up to ten rounds.

Points to note

After a few weeks of practice, hold the legs-up final pose for far longer, for greater impact.

How it works

- This is the classic yogic crunch, which tautens the tummy.
- Tones liver, encouraging stored fat release.

Other benefits

- Boosts digestion, ups nutrient absorption, thus managing hunger.
- Trims hips and thighs.
- Increases stamina.
- Controls diabetes.

NAUKASANA (BOAT POSE, SEATED VERSION)

Method

- To be done seated.
- Follow instructions in previous exercise, up to the point where you lift legs in air.
- Then, exhaling gently, straighten both legs, so that they are parallel to the ground or higher. This provides more of a challenge to the abdomen. You may place feet on a table in front, if you wish, though that reduces the impact somewhat.
- Hold the pose, breathing normally. Inhale, dropping feet back to the ground.
- Do up to ten times.
- After a few weeks, increase duration in the final pose as well the number, for actual impact.

How it works and other benefits

As above, with more enhanced benefits and greater tone.

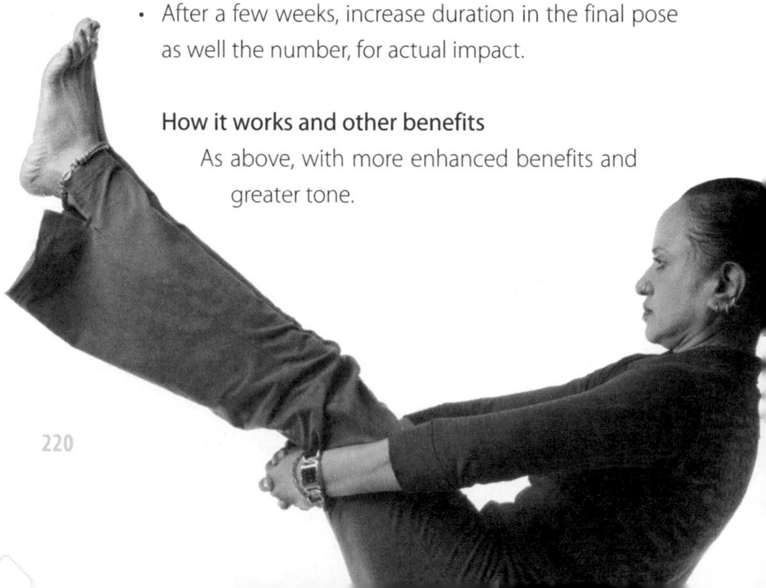

NAUKA SANCHALANASANA (BOAT ROWING POSE)

Method

- Sit sideways on a chair, so that the back rest is on your right (or left).
- Place both palms in front of you to hold the chair edge, (as shown in the picture below).
- Inhale, tilting back deeply.
- Hold the pose, breathing evenly.
- Ensure your feet remain flat on the ground. This gives a better support plus enhances the stretch.
- Exhale, release, straightening body back to starting position.
- Repeat a few times.

Points to note

- After sufficient practice, you may hold your breath for a few seconds in the final pose. However, remember that breath retention is contraindicated for cardiac and circulatory problems.
- The time in the final pose must also be extended for added impact. You may

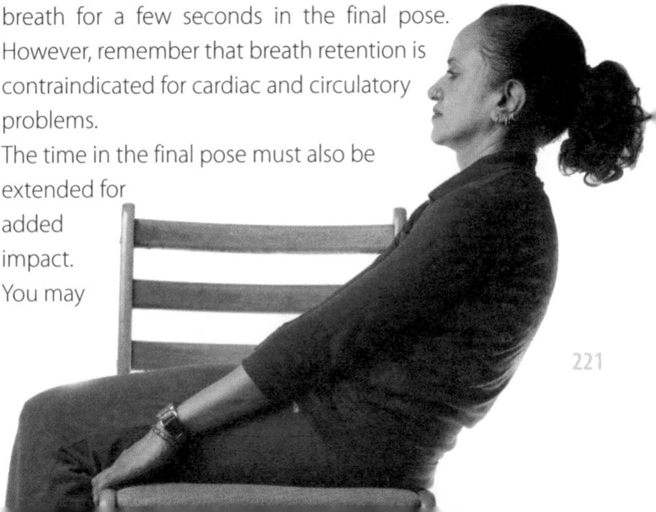

increase it from fifteen seconds up to thirty or more, after sufficient and regular practice. But in that case, continue normal breathing.

How it works

- This acts like a passive, but effective crunch, toning your belly.
- Works on lower abs.

Other benefits

- This opens the chest, boosting respiration.
- Uplifts mood.
- Works the spine.
- Legs get toned due to the resistance induced by the tilt.

BHARADWAJASANA (SAGE BHARADWAJA POSE)

Method

- Sit on a chair.
- Keep knees together.
- Inhale, passing right hand over back rest, and placing left hand gently on right knee.
- Exhale, twist firmly to the right, to look over the right shoulder.
- Hold the pose, breathing normally.
- Repeat thrice.
- Rest, to repeat for the left side.

Points to note

- Holding the final pose longer will enhance benefits.
- Remember to hold the stomach muscles in while doing the pose.

How it works

- It trims the entire abdomen.
- It squeezes the liver into releasing fat.
- It helps control stress and diabetes, both implicated strongly in belly fat.

Other benefits

- Gives a gentle, yet definitive spinal traction, preventing all spinal problems.
- Is therapeutic in neck pain.
- Boosts respiration.
- Is a cure-all pose, toning immunity too.
- Facial and neck muscles are also worked out, making your skin glow.
- Is anti-ageing.

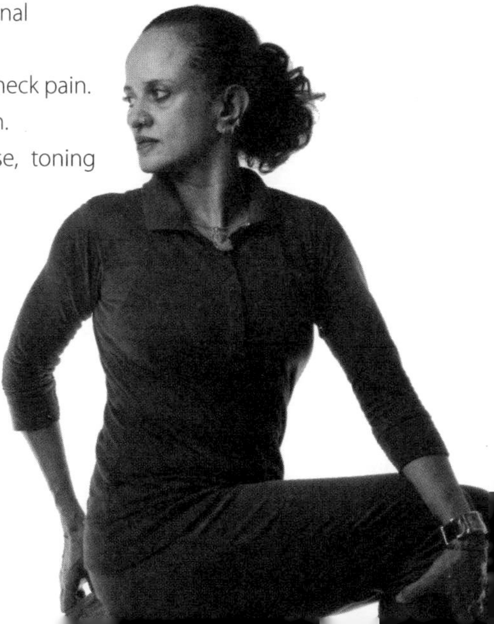

KATI CHAKRASANA (HIP CIRCLE)

Method

- Stand up straight.
- Feet must be together or slightly apart. The latter is advised for those whose balance is shaky.
- Place hands on waist.
- Inhale. Exhaling, gently jut your hip to the right.
- Exhale, move hip backwards, jutting it out behind.
- Inhale, move it to left.
- Exhale, move it out in front.
- This completes one circle. Do five to ten circles.

Points to note

- In each movement, only the hips must move, the feet must remain where placed.
- You may do this slowly, drawing a clockwise circle with your hips thrice. Essentially you are doing a gentle version of a belly dance, drawing a circle with your hips in the clockwise direction.
- After you have gained mastery over the movement, you may learn to do it in an anti-clockwise direction too, repeating an equal number of circles in either direction.

How it works

- It trims abdominal fat all around.

- Encourages the liver to release fat.
- Boosts digestion.
- Spikes metabolism.

Other benefits

- Peps you up by removing stiffness and lethargy from the body.
- Works out legs, toning them.
- Improves limb-brain coordination.
- Is therapeutic in diabetes.

What else?

- All tummy trimmers are also effective in **diabetic treatment**, because they impact the pancreas positively.
- They are also super **stress-busters**. They massage the stress or adrenal glands, helping to rejuvenate them.
- They help tone the rest of the body too, since you need to work out connected parts to trim fat at the abdomen.

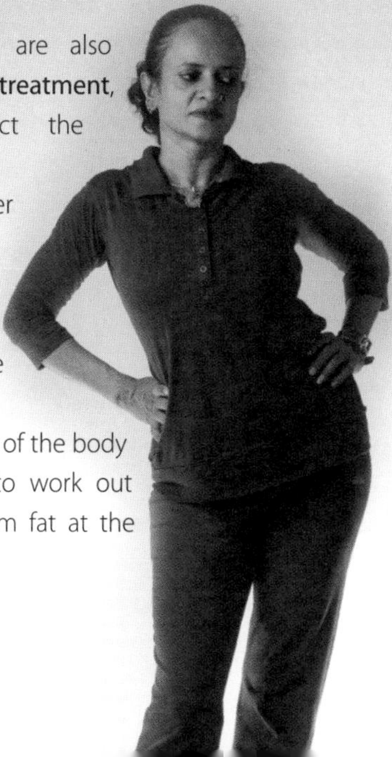

This book has modified classic yoga poses that can easily be done at your workplace. The idea is to retain the basic structure of the pose but adapt it to an office set-up so the movement may be done discreetly yet effectively.

The effect of such practices may not be as potent as that of classical yoga done on a mat, but it is immediate nevertheless. So, if health is your choice, then keep this book as a reference guide for yoga at work, and also enrol in a yoga class which you may attend at least a few days in a week. This will power your desk-top yoga further.

The reasons why it is urgent to practice these poses have already been emphasised in each chapter. Here we discuss how you may prepare your own yogic regimen from this book.

HOW TO USE THIS BOOK

- Remember to do some warm-ups, like shoulder shrugs, ankle rotations, hand and wrist rotations and finger stretches (also explained in the book; you may also access the desk-top warm-up chart — Page 232 — for this). This will prevent unnecessary cramps, to which those who have body stiffness are prone. This is common with those who have circulatory problems, diabetes (also pre-diabetes) or nutrition deficiency.

- If you do get a cramp, it is not an earth-shattering event. It merely is a symptom of one or the other cause which we just listed above. You must try to factor in magnesium-rich foods like nuts, dark green vegetables and leafy greens, brown rice, whole grains (not refined or white rice or packed atta). If a cramp occurs, wait for it to pass by keeping the body still. It is just an indication that the muscle you activated is not releasing energy fast enough. This also decreases once your body gets flexible and your muscles become more active and supple.
- Choose the chapter of particular relevance to you (if you have diabetes, for instance, you may wish to start with tummy tucking), and repeat a few times during the day. Use the warm-up chart before such a practice.
- Once you have established a routine of warm-ups and

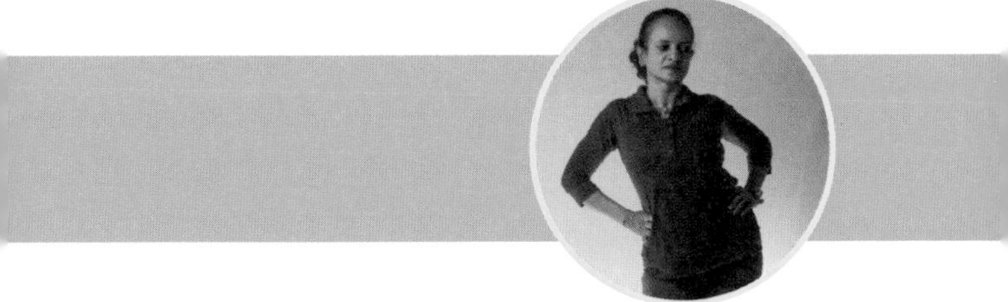

the chosen chart in your daily life, start introducing one of the sadhana charts, either the long (Page 234) or the short one (Page 232), depending on how your day unfolds.

- Once you have got a particular problem under control (such as a back pain or high blood pressure or depression) you may drop that particular exercise set and practice only either one of the sadhana charts. However, revert to the special ailment exercise once a week to ensure that you do not suffer a relapse.
- You can scan the charts, pinning it near your desk. However, my advice is: don't be too dependent on a chart. Once you practice regularly, just remember the flow naturally. I have known my students to skip practice just because they did not have the chart around on that particular day!
- Ideally you should create your own chart of practices from this book, promising yourself that you will run through them during your working day. A set of ten to twelve practices is sufficient to ensure complete health. Unless you have a specific health issue, do not create a chart that focuses on only one body part or health gain. Create a practice regimen that includes the entire body.
- When you start on this programme, you may start with just a few rounds. We have deliberately refrained from suggesting how many you may do: this will depend on how much time you can spare at work. However, as you advance in practice, and learn to regularise it, increase the number of rounds substantially, from ten to even thirty. This is because when you move a

particular muscle group in a certain way or pose, after just six weeks it gets used to the pose. So, even though health is assured, if you are looking for cosmetic value from such a practice (as in greater muscle tone, more structuring and body-shaping) it is crucial to prevent muscular 'boredom' and keep upping the challenge.

- If you are doing challenging rounds, ideally you must also factor in a cool-down period. This is crucial for maximising the benefits. In case you don't have time, it is better that you do less of the main poses to accommodate the cool-down instead of skipping it altogether. To jump from a vigorous exercise into another activity means the body does not get to remove the blood lactate load from the arteries. This means you may feel irritated, oversensitive or fatigued later on. The corpse pose (shavasana) — lying back with feet apart, hands slightly away from the body, palms facing upwards, with both eyes shut — is the perfect cool-down pose. However that may not be practical in a formal space like an office. Instead, the practitioner may remain seated in a relaxed fashion, with eyes shut, till the breath returns to normal. This is a perfect substitute as a cool down pose.
- Though a normal strenuous round of yoga requires you to take a two to four hour gap between meal time and practice, these poses do not require you to take such a long gap — a half-hour to one hour gap should be fine since these are modified poses. However, try

not to do them immediately after a meal. Position them just before a meal, if crunched for time.

- Fix a particular time, ideally before lunch or tea break for this programme. This will ensure that you will never miss it. Practising erratically can make you miss the practice.
- At least thrice during the week try to do a full set of classic poses, ideally in a yoga class, for a minimum of half an hour at least. This is crucial to complement the effort you make at office.
- Once you regularise your practice, advance to include a fixed pranayama and meditation practice into your day. Ideally, you must do your meditation and pranayama at home before coming to work. Then you can relegate your yogic stretches to office.
- Try to get an office buddy to participate or partner you in this regimen. This will keep your motivation high, and ensure regularity.
- Ideally yoga must be done in a meditative fashion. So don't try to juggle these stretches while talking on the phone or while punching your keyboard. Only when the mind focuses on the muscle being worked out does it result in good health. This is true even for gym-based exercises.
- And for those of you who are convinced about the value of this workout but feel constrained by certain social inhibitions, I can assure that it is more than likely that your colleagues will also, after some initial curiosity

and bantering, take to it. This incorporation inevitably happens, especially if you are able to convey the idea that it is cool to do yoga at office, as indeed it is. In Japan and the US, the more progressive companies offer stretch breaks. Companies are promoting the idea of healthy practices at the workplace because it increases productivity and reduces absenteeism!

- Some facts about contraindications — it is best to observe them, especially if you are a casual or infrequent practitioner. However, if you are regular practitioner, then as soon as you have got your problem under control (spinal problems, diabetes, blood pressure, respiratory problems) and are sure that it is unlikely to erupt or you no longer fear a relapse, you can incorporate even a contraindicated pose. Ideally, if you have joined a yoga class we suggest you check with your instructor as to when you may incorporate such contraindicated poses into your sadhana.
- Where we have mentioned some poses as stimulating, it means the mind becomes alert. Such poses are best avoided just before sleep time, since they will keep you wide awake (chest openers, hyperventilating pranayamas are some examples).
- Finally, regularity is more important than a lengthy but sporadic practice. So, try to start off with a fifteen-minute practice that is regularly done instead of doing an hour-long chart that is done weekly.

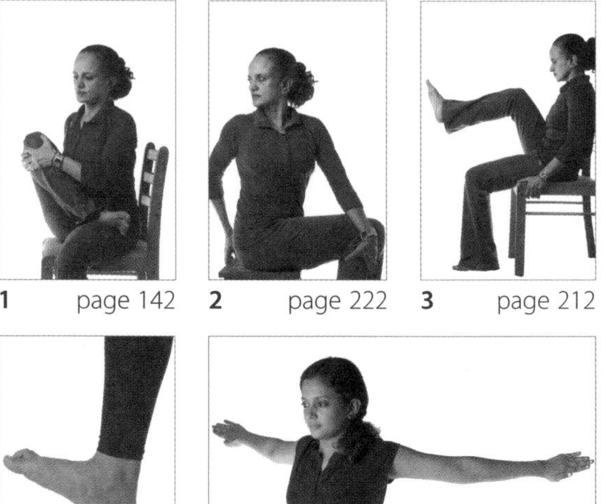

1 page 142 **2** page 222 **3** page 212

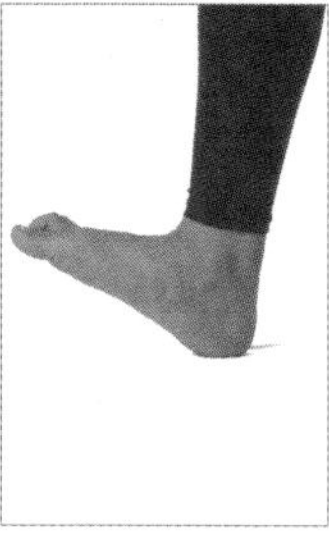

6 page 16

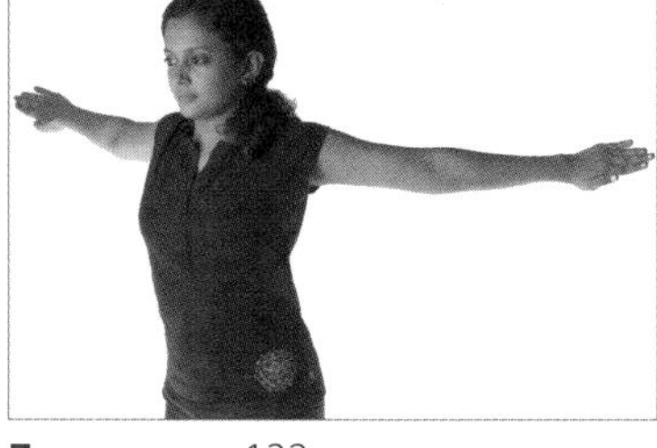

7 page 132

WARM-UP CHART

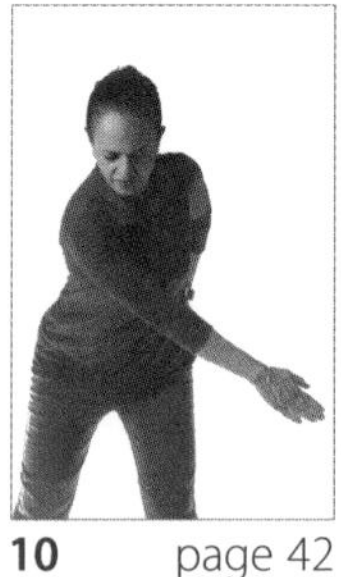

10 page 42

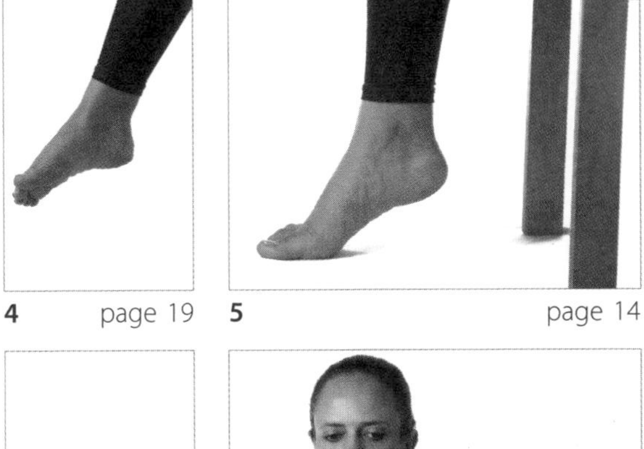

4 page 19 **5** page 14

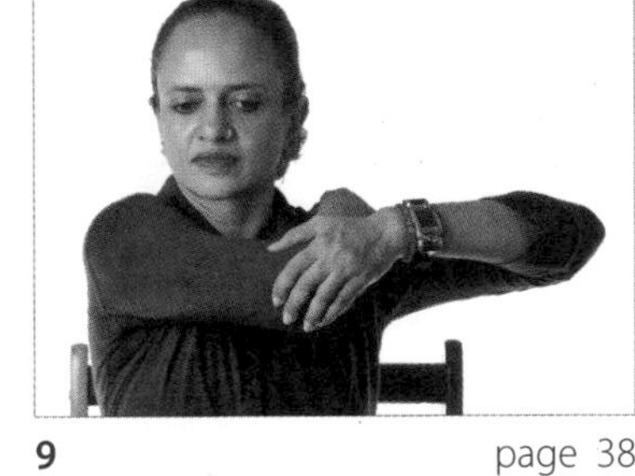

8 page 133 **9** page 38

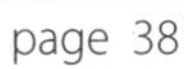

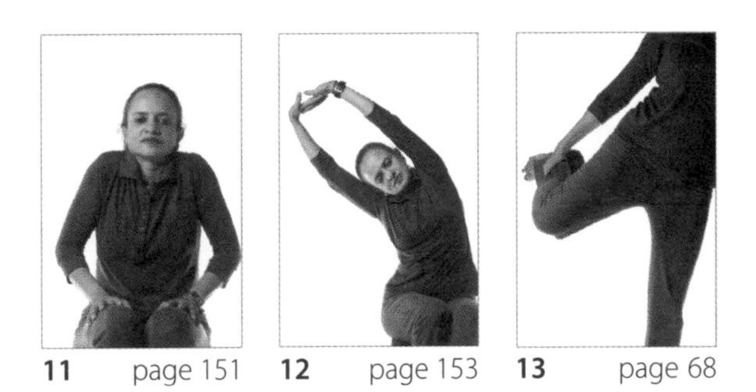

11 page 151 **12** page 153 **13** page 68

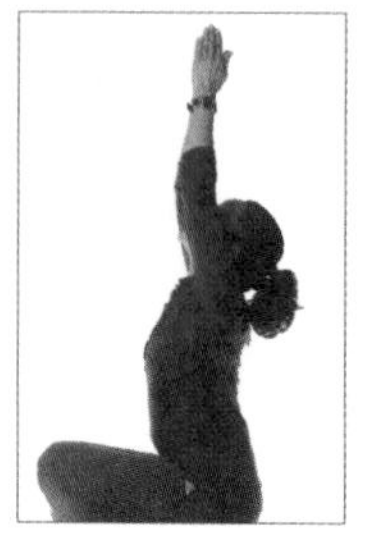

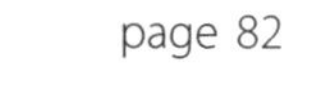

1 page 82

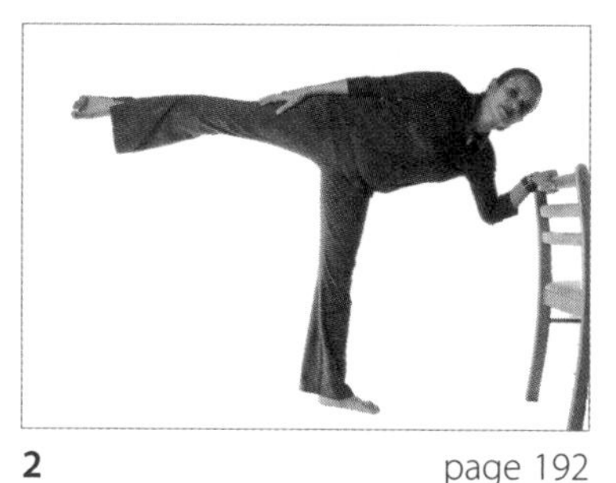

2 page 192

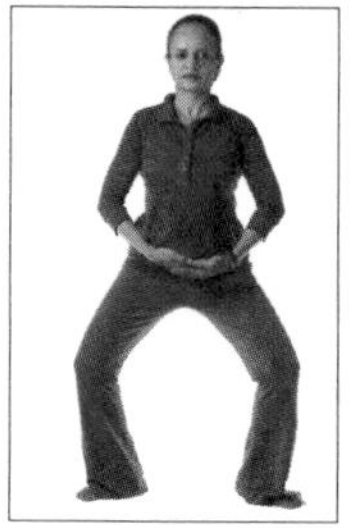

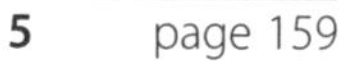

5 page 159

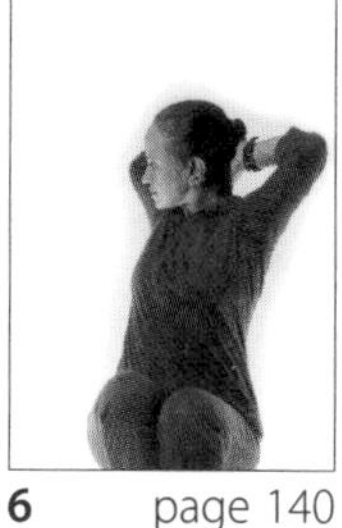

6 page 140

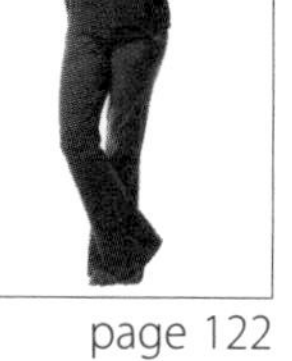

7 page 122

PRACTICE CHART

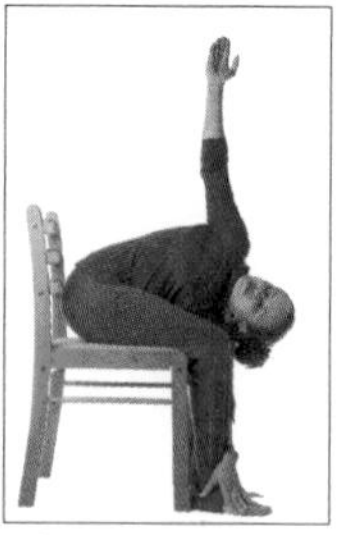

10 page 110

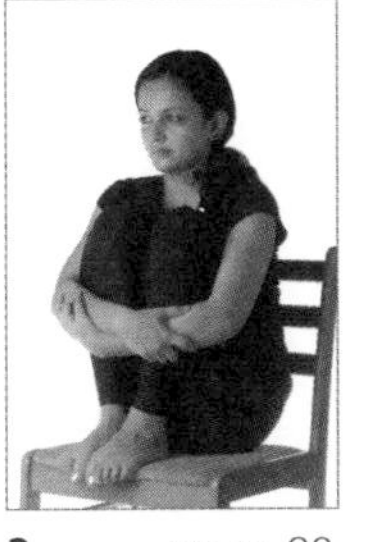

3 page 90

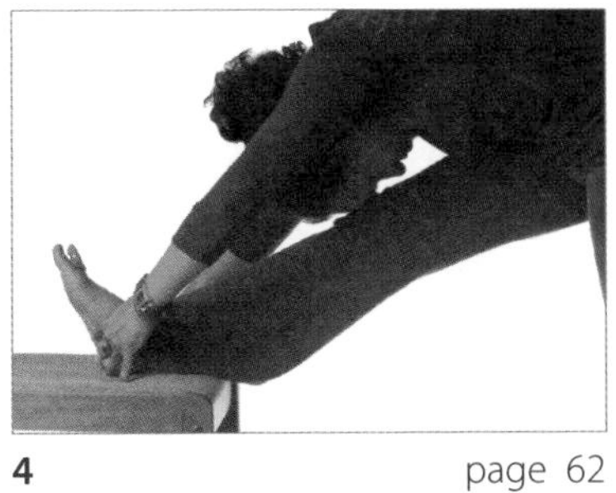

4 page 62

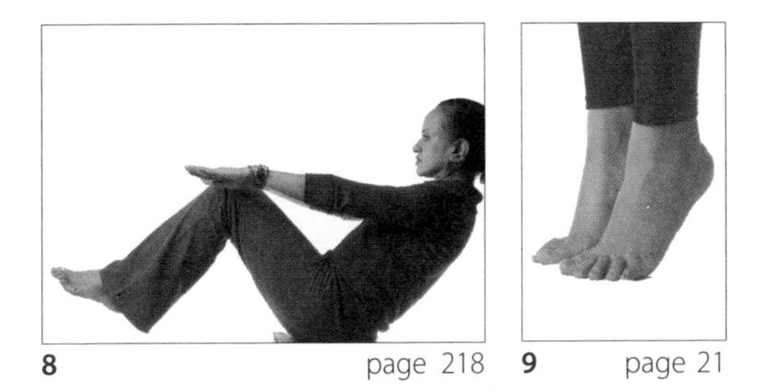

8 page 218

9 page 21

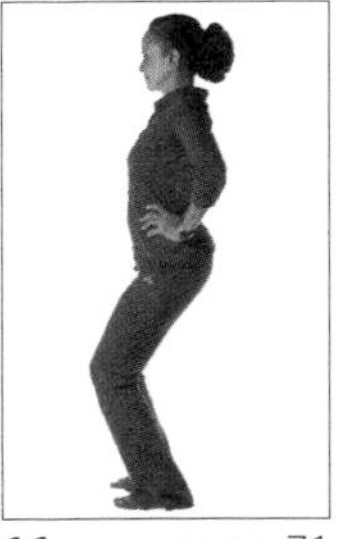

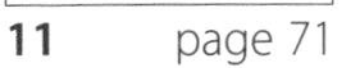

11 page 71

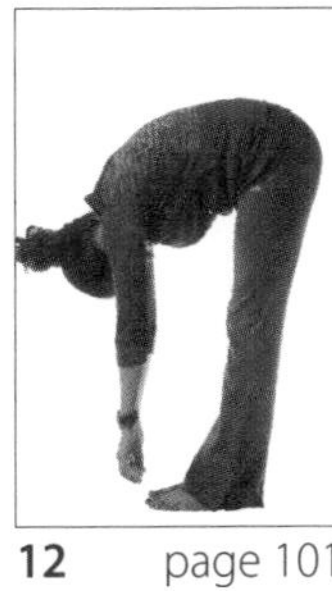

12 page 101

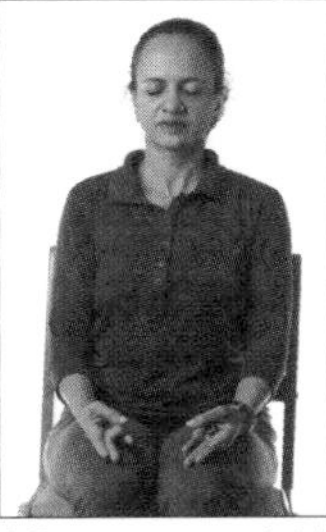

13 page 144

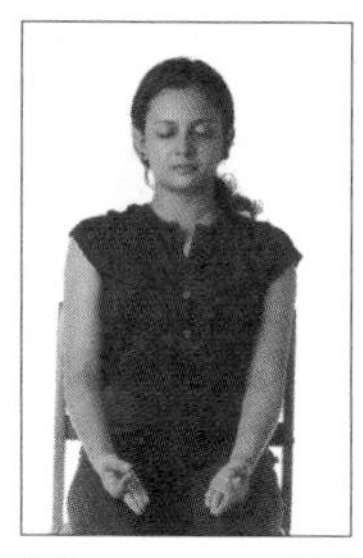

14 page 116

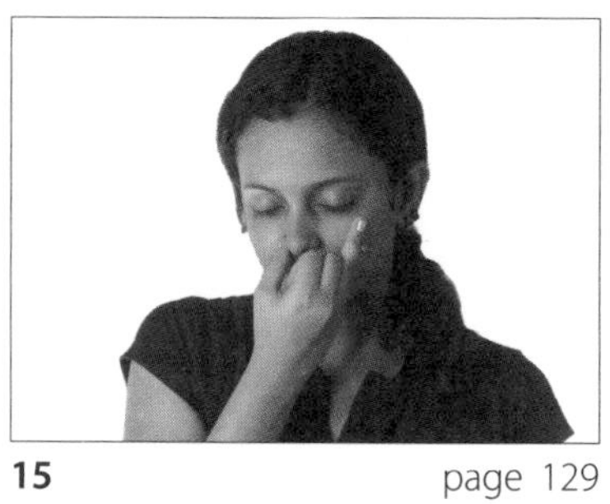

15 page 129

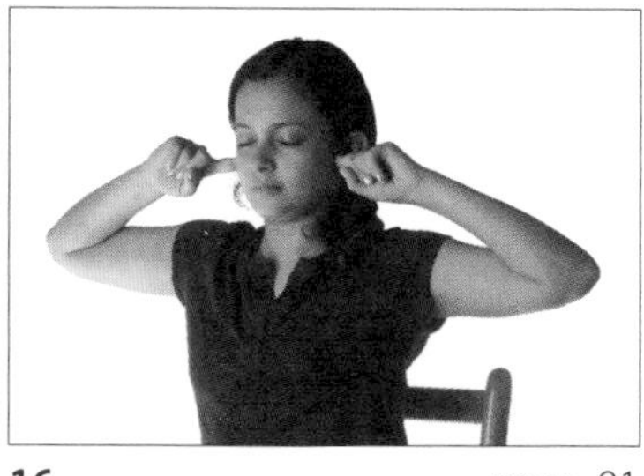

16 page 91